VEGETARIAN HIGH-FIBRE COOKING

A collection of delicious recipes to inspire you to a healthier
way of eating.

About the Author

Janette Marshall was, until recently, deputy editor of *Here's Health*, the
leading magazine in the field of natural health. She is now a freelance
author and journalist in all areas of alternative lifestyles, healthy living
and consumer issues. Her previous books include *The Wholefood Party
Book* and *The Wholefood Cookery Course* which she wrote with Sarah
Bounds.

VEGETARIAN HIGH-FIBRE COOKING

by
JANETTE MARSHALL

THORSONS PUBLISHING GROUP
Wellingborough, Northamptonshire
·
Rochester, Vermont

First published in 1983 as
High-Fibre Cooking

This revised, reset, colour-illustrated
edition first published 1987

© JANETTE MARSHALL 1987

British Library Cataloguing in Publication Data

Marshall, Janette
[High-fibre cooking]. Vegetarian high-fibre
cooking.
1. Vegetarian cookery   2. High-fibre diet
I. [High-fibre cooking]   II. Title
641.5'636   TX837

ISBN 0-7225-1529-4

Printed in Great Britain

2 4 6 8 10 9 7 5 3 1

CONTENTS

This book is dedicated to better health.

INTRODUCTION

By now just about everyone has heard of fibre and has some idea that it is important and necessary for health. If you ask most people to name some high-fibre foods the first words that fall from their lips are 'bran' and 'baked beans' yet, since they were popularized at the beginning of the 1980s, a lot has happened to increase our knowledge and introduce us to different types of fibre found in other foods apart from beans and bran.

For anyone interested in their health this will be exciting news because it brings more information from which to make enlightened food choices, and for anyone bored with bran it gives a far wider choice of high-fibre foods. However, it doesn't mean that bran is now out of fashion or no longer thought to be effective. It just means that we now know more about the way in which fibre works as a preventive medicine, or as a curative one where health problems exist.

PART 1

1.

WHY WE NEED FIBRE

For a long time fibre was regarded as useless. It was described as roughage and because it passed through the body without apparently giving us any calories for energy, or nutrients such as vitamins and minerals, it was thought to be unimportant. Well into the 1950s dietitians were being taught that roughage was over-rated and of no consequence.

It was not until 1969 that the surgeon Mr Denis Burkitt linked common Western diseases such as cancer of the colon, coronary heart disease, diverticulitis, diabetes, haemorrhoids and appendicitis with a lack of fibre in the diet that medical opinion started to change. As a medical missionary he had seen few of these diseases in Africa and he suggested that the high level of fibre in the unrefined diets of African villagers protected them.

His interest had been aroused by reading the work of the late Surgeon Captain Peter Cleave. In an obituary to Surgeon Captain Cleave, Denis Burkitt said, 'Although a few others have also recognized that these diseases were characteristically western, Cleave was the first to accumulate, through much painstaking and persistent work, evidence not only incriminating diet as a causative factor, but putting particular blame on the refining of carbohydrate foods with resultant excess of sugar consumption and a deficiency of fibre intake.'

Much of the pioneering work by these men started with observations that the frequency and volume of bowel movements of African people living on an unrefined diet of mainly grains, fruit and vegetables greatly exceeded those of people eating a typical Western diet. It was also noticed that the high fibre content of their diet speeded up the transit time, eliminating toxic waste far more quickly.

Constipation

It was obvious that there were benefits to be gained by people in the West who may rely on habitual use of laxatives because, for a start, increasing fibre could cure constipation which is one of the commonest complaints in Western civilization, costing the National Health Service more than £8 million in 1985 for laxative prescriptions in England alone; and this figure does not include the vast amount spent over the counter by those who buy their own purgatives.

Habitual reliance on laxatives can result in a bowel which is unable to function without this stimulation, and the fluid stool that results can deplete the body of salts, vitamins and minerals and result, eventually in damage to the colon that might require surgery.

Acceptance of a small bowel motion once or twice a week could be equally potentially dangerous and the physical straining involved in evacuating hard stools in constipation can lead to other problems such as haemorrhoids, varicose veins and even hiatus hernia.

The longer time it takes for waste products to travel through a sluggish system also means that toxic waste products are in contact with the digestive tract for a longer time, which means there is a greater risk of reabsorbing dangerous toxins. A high-fibre diet can bring the transit time from two weeks in an elderly person or three days in a healthy younger person nearer to the 1½ days on the unrefined African diet.

Haemorrhoids, Varicose veins, Hiatus hernia

These three conditions are common among people eating a typical refined diet and have been grouped together because they can be the direct result of constipation. For a long time haemorrhoids were thought to be anal varicose veins, but now they are thought to be a prolapse of part of the anal region which is full of blood vessel caused by straining at stool.

Veins are the vessels that return blood to the heart after the oxygen has been delivered to body cells via the arteries. The veins contain valves to stop the blood flowing backwards against the flow of gravity which it is likely to do in the legs. During abdominal straining in constipation the blood is forced to flow back down the legs causing the veins to stretch. Eventually the veins will not be able to function properly and varicose veins will develop. This will happen more easily in people with an hereditary disposition.

Hiatus hernias can be another direct result of straining and they are prevalent in middle-aged people who eat a low-fibre diet. The hernia results when pressure builds up in the abdomen and the top of the stomach is forced through a hole in the diaphragm through which the digestive tract passes.

Diverticulitis

This disease began to appear at the beginning of the 1900s and by 1960 was the most common disease of the colon in the West. More than one third of people are thought to have diverticula by the time they are 40 and the incidence increases with age. Diverticula are pocket like pouches in the wall of the colon caused by a build up of pressure in the colon.

The pressure build up occurs when the regular waves that are needed to propel a soft faecal mass along the colon are not enough to propel the hard faeces which are typical of a low-fibre diet. The colon walls have to contract harder and this causes areas of pressure to occur in the gaps between the hard waste matter. In these areas pressure builds up and causes small 'blow outs' of the colon wall, producing pockets called diverticula in a way that has been likened to the bulges of the inner tube through the outer wall of a tyre.

Before the discovery of the importance of fibre, people with diverticulitis were put on a diet free from roughage because it was thought that this would 'aggravate' the gut. Now it is realized that the missing fibre contributed to the disease, a high-fibre diet is prescribed for diverticula patients, although it cannot cure the problem because it is not a reversible condition. However, it can remove constipation, prevent further occurrences and reduce the colic like pains associated with the disease.

Appendictis

This is a health problem rarely found among people of Africa, but like heart disease it is something that such people develop when they move to urbanized environments with a Western diet. It is a disease with substantial evidence to show that a high-fibre diet lessens its chances of occurring. For example, the number of cases in England and Wales dropped between 1971 and 1975 and reports in the British medical press have shown the decrease to be concurrent with an increase in the consumption of wholemeal bread, fresh fruit and vegetables.

Appendicitis occurs when the appendix, a blind-ended tube of about two inches (5cm) in length found at the beginning of the large intestine, becomes blocked and subsequently infected. The blockage is usually caused by a small lump of hard faeces, typical of a low-fibre diet. If the faeces are soft there is less likelihood of an appendix blockage and infection.

Gallstones

Along with appendicitis, gallstones are the commonest cause of abdominal operations and nearly 50 per cent of women will have gallstones by the time they are in their 80s (men are half as likely to get gallstones). Some gallstones are pure cholesterol and most are about 70 per cent cholesterol.

They form when the bile acids (produced to digest fatty foods) are super-saturated with cholesterol for various reasons and the risks increase with age, obesity and oestrogen treatment, but on the plus side they are found less often in populations eating a high-fibre diet which has been demonstrated in studies of British vegetarians who show far less than the average incidence of gallstones.

To induce gallstones in animals they have to be fed a lot of low-fibre carbohydrate foods, such as sugar, and research has shown that such gallstones can be prevented by adding fibre to the animals' diets — or even just allowing them to eat their bedding straw!

Changing the diets of humans from the typical British diet to a diet high in unrefined carbohydrates and slightly lower in calories than the average has tipped the balance effectively away from bile that contains the amount of cholesterol likely to cause gallstones to healthy non-saturated bile.

Adding bran has done the trick in diet trials because it speeds transit time. This helps prevent certain bacterial conditions in the colon occurring where a secondary type of super-saturated bile acid is formed from the original bile. Prolonged fasting also allows bile to stagnate in the gallbladder, where it is produced, thus encouraging stone formation and giving another good reason why we should eat a good breakfast, according to Dr Kenneth Heaton, an authority on gallstones and fibre.

Diabetes

During digestion carbohydrates are broken down into their constituent sugars which are absorbed into the bloodstream to provide energy. It is the job of insulin to make this energy available to the body and when diabetes occurs there is a lack of effective insulin. Without insulin sugar builds up in the blood, effectively starving the body of energy.

In the past it was thought that diabetics had to avoid carbohydrate and obtain as much of their energy as possible from fat. But with the discovery that unrefined carbohydrate foods produce a very steady release of energy into the bloodstream and do not make sudden demands for insulin, like sugar and refined foods made from it do, then the balance of diabetics' diets has changed. Now wholemeal bread and pasta, brown rice, cereals, grains and starchy vegetables and fruits are on the menu for diabetics because the effect of fibre is to iron out the ups and downs of diabetics' blood sugar levels.

The cereal fibres with their bran contents seem to help diabetics keep their fasting blood glucose levels stable and the gummy fibre in beans and oats reduces immediate rises after a meal. Diabetics, like everyone else who eats a diet high in unrefined carbohydrates, are benefiting from the steady, slow release of energy from these foods. Probably more than everyone else they need to also watch their weight — and, of course, they need to avoid sugar and sugary food (which we should all be doing).

Obesity

Many maturity-onset diabetics find they also have a weight problem and if they switch to a high-fibre diet this very often sorts itself out. In the same way a high-fibre diet can help people lose weight as many who have tried the *F-Plan Diet* or who have switched to a wholefood diet can witness. The greater bulk of food leads to more chewing and a feeling of satiety, which is enhanced because fibre keeps food in the stomach for longer and results in a slower release of energy.

For those who are actually slimming unrefined foods also contain more vitamins and minerals than many mono-diets would. When reducing quantity of food it is especially important to maintain, or improve, quality and this helps prevent the 'lows' that might otherwise occur on a slimming diet. It also prevents another bugbear of reducing diets — constipation which makes the dieter feel worse, especially when niggly and hungry! Adding bran to food is also useful if it is a low-fibre diet.

There has also been a suggestion that a proportion of calories remain undigested when the diet is high in fibre, although there is no evidence to support the idea that fibre has a negative calorie effect, however, carbohydrate foods are less likely to be deposited as fat than fatty foods.

All good reducing diets are based on high-fibre unrefined carbohydrate regimens which no longer rule out the spaghetti and spuds that the old-fashioned low-carbohydrate high-protein diets did. The real benefits of this pattern of eating is that it is a long-term, sustainable form of eating, unlike diets which impose an unnatural pattern of eating which, when abandoned after a diet, leads to regaining the weight along with the old, bad eating habits.

Coronary Heart Disease

There are many risk factors involved in heart disease, from being male to smoking, lack of exercise, raised blood-pressure, eating a diet too high in saturated fats and even being overweight and diabetic — two conditions which we have seen fibre can help. Increasingly heart disease has been linked with the typical high-fat, high-sugar and therefore low, unrefined carbohydrate and low-fibre diet.

It is in the risk area of fats that fibre has been seen to be especially helpful in two ways. Firstly its presence in the diet has been shown to reduce the amount of serum cholesterol, that is the type of cholesterol that is circulating in the bloodstream, and is liable to be deposited as plaque, which silts up the arteries.

This narrows the passages through which the blood flows and so prevents the heart receiving all the blood, and thus oxygen, it needs to work efficiently. The arteries may even silt up completely, or a blood clot may lodge in a narrowed artery preventing oxygenated blood reaching the heart muscle and if the supply is cut off completely a heart attack happens.

Not only can fibre help reduce the amount of cholesterol but it can also alter the type of cholesterol in a beneficial way. A type of cholesterol called high density lipoprotein (HDL) which is thought to be protective against heart disease, has been seen to increase in high-fibre eaters and low density lipoprotein, thought to be harmful, has been seen to decrease. There is also evidence to suggest that fibre may make blood less likely to clot.

High Blood-Pressure

As we have seen this is a risk factor in heart disease and is usually found in middle-aged and older people, or pregnant women. Interestingly Western vegetarians, along with the rural Africans studied by the fibre pioneers, have been shown to have lower blood-pressure than those who eat a meat-based diet that is low in fibre. (Other dietary modifications such as reducing salt and keeping weight in check also have good effect.) Fibre may also influence hormones that cause high blood-pressure.

Cancer of the Colon

Many foods, both natural and processed or manufactured foods containing artificial additives, contain chemicals that are potentially carcinogenic, and constipation, due to lack of fibre in the diet, means that the colon and rectum are exposed for longer periods to toxic residues in faeces.

As yet no one chemical or substance has been linked positively to cancers of the bowel, but the fact that African populations show far lower incidence of these cancers than people on a Western diet has suggested that high-fibre diets, in reducing transit time and diluting faecal contents, reduce the risk of exposure to these unidentified carcinogens.

There may also be an hereditary influence in that some people have a genetic predisposition enabling them to handle poisons better, or making them more susceptible to their effects. Diet may also have a general influence in providing the necessary raw materials to enable the body to repair damaged cells and reverse the many-stepped process towards cancer cells being produced.

For example, choline-deficient (part of the B vitamin complex) and vitamin C deficient diets have been shown in rats to inhibit their ability to make repairs to lesions. Feeding them known dietary carcinogens along with large doses of vitamin C has proved vitamin C to be protective.

Levels of both fat and fibre in the diet have been seen to influence the conversion of bacteria which live in the gut and are essential for digestion, into harmful or potentially carcinogenic 'faecal mutagens' which may be a risk factor in cancer of the large bowel. Experiments have shown that raising the level of fibre in particular not only produces larger bowel movements but also movements with significantly fewer mutagens.

Other research has shown that patients with polyps in the colon (which may, in some cases, develop into cancers) also have high levels of mutagens but that supplements of vitamins C and E may slightly reduce the risk of further polyps developing after surgery.

Studies on animals have also suggested that providing more calcium than is normally present on a standard diet gives some protection against the toxic effect of bile acids on the cells of the intestines. An unrefined diet will provide both fibre to bind with bile acids and calcium which is protective. High-fibre diets also mean there is less room for fatty foods which can increase health risks.

Breast Cancer

Breast cancer has been linked with diet in various ways, one of which involves fibre as a preventive. Recent medical research has come round to the long-held naturopathic view that women's breasts take up toxic wastes that have been reabsorbed into the bloodstream from waste matter that can linger in the intestine.

This is supported by the association noted between constipation and lumpy breasts, cystic breast disease and cancer. Cystic disease has been seen to improve when constipation is relieved.

Lumpy breasts can also be caused by changes in hormone balance which are sometimes brought about by high-fat levels in the diet. The hormone progesterone may also bind with chemical substances in caffeine to produce lumpy breasts.

Although the interplay of fibre, gut bacteria and absorption of carcinogenic toxins from waste in the gut is still being researched the indications are that vegetarian women on a high-fibre diet are less likely to have breast disease. This is because the fibre may induce production of beneficial oestrogen hormones (usually found in higher levels in vegetarian women) which are protective.

Women with severe mastalgia and breast swelling are also known to find relief on high-fibre diets. The role of vitamin A and calcium, found in carrots and dark green vegetables, may also be linked to vegetarians' protection.

Lung Cancer
A 10 year study in Holland which scrutinized the diet and medical histories of 1000 middle-aged men confirmed that low-fibre intake increased the risk of heart disease and other diseases associated with low-fibre intake. It also highlighted the less well known link of low-fibre diet and deaths from cancer. Surprisingly, lung cancer occurred more in the low-fibre intake group where the men's diet lacked beta-carotene (which is made into vitamin A in the body) found in carrots and dark green vegetables — also good sources of fibre.

Teeth and Gums
Teeth and gums, as well as general health, will benefit from a high-fibre wholefood diet. The fresh fruit and vegetables, wholemeal bread, grains and pulses mean less room for sticky cakes and sweets which provide sugar to stick to the teeth and feed the bacteria that produce

the acid to attack enamel and cause caries. The chewing and crunching of unrefined foods also keeps the mouth clean and fresh and helps ensure that only the right kind of bacteria take up residence!

2.

WHAT IS FIBRE?

Fibre is found in carbohydrate foods. These are the starches that give us energy when they are broken down into their constituent sugars during the process of digestion. Fibre is found in greater quantities in unrefined carbohydrate foods such as wholemeal bread and flour, brown rice and beans, cereals, lentils, fruit and vegetables. From this list you will see that fibre comes from plant foods.

It is part of the plant's polysaccharide, or starch energy store, and in man the starch is digested to give energy, but the non-starch polysaccharide — the fibre — is not digested. Until recently it was thought that all the starch was digested in the small intestine and then the fibre component passed to the large intestine where it was fermented by bacteria and then excreted.

But now it has been discovered that some starch in processed foods is resistant to the body's digestive enzymes. This is called *resistant starch* and *partially resistant starch* and, in common with fibre, they are not digested; although unlike fibre they are not part of the plant's cell wall.

There has been some suggestion that resistant starch could be classified with dietary fibre to produce the fibre counts that you see on nutritional labels of food products, but because it is not part of the cell wall this has been resisted and scientists have pointed out that it might be an important food component in its own right — which has yet to be discovered.

Initial experiments have shown that starch which is resistant to digestion is found in foods such as raw potato and under-ripe banana, and some starch in grains and beans is partially resistant. Other experiments have shown that food processing from freeze drying to autoclaving can affect how much of the starch is available for the body to digest.

It seems that freshly cooked foods are completely digested but the longer food is left, held warm or reheated the more resistant starch is produced. For example, a potato cooked and reheated four times will produce five grams of resistant starch per 100 grams.

Similarly, finely milled wholemeal flour will be more accessible to the body for digestion than more coarsely milled flour and when white flour or bread is autoclaved at very high temperatures, up to 10–15 per cent of resistant starch can be produced in bread. It has even been suggested that up to 20 per cent could be produced to make a very 'high-fibre' bread that would supply all 'dietary fibre' needs, but this is as 'unnatural' as adding bran without reforming the rest of the diet.

However, resistant starch is not yet classified as dietary fibre and if it were to be allowed food manufacturers could use it to undermine the true value of dietary fibre as a food component. It is likely that a method for analysis and labelling standards will be drawn up by the Ministry of Agriculture which includes the 'sum non-starch polysaccharides' and does not include the resistant starch.

This might be included in the bread and flour regulations which do not contain reference to fibre limits for different types of bread at the moment. It might also provide some surprises when new methods of analysis show that foods previously regarded as high-fibre might not be so high in true fibre, but may contain a large proportion of resistant starch. Cornflakes, for example, currently appearing in literature as containing 10 grams of fibre per 100 grams may be nearer to one gram of fibre (the remainder being resistant starch) if resistant starch is not included in future in dietary fibre counts.

How much resistant starch our food contains is therefore very much in the hands of food processors and manufacturers and, for this reason, there needs to be more research into the effects of this starch on our health. For the time being we can still think of fibre as the plant's cell wall and if you imagine a plant cell wall to be like a cardboard box the fibre is the equivalent of the sides of the box. Pile several boxes on top of each other and you have a simplified illustration of the way the fibre in plant cell walls enables the plant to stay upright.

Animal cells do not contain fibre, but that doesn't mean they are always falling over! Humans and animals are kept upright by their skeletons. Muscles are attached to the bones to move the body about. The basic difference is important because it highlights the fact that fibre is only available from plant foods. Meat, fish and dairy products are devoid of fibre.

Not all plants contain the same amount of fibre, and the structure of plant cell walls changes as the plant matures and grows. The cell wall itself is made up of cellulose, hemicelluloses, pectins, gums, mucilages (from seeds and seaweeds) and lignins which encrust the outside of cell walls in mature and woody plants.

Types of Fibre
There are two classifications of fibre that describe what it can do for is; **soluble** and **insoluble.**

Soluble fibre such as the betaglucan gums in beans and in oats and the gels in pectin have an important role in helping to lower serum cholesterol levels — which bran cannot do. They bind and remove bile acids preventing fats such as cholesterol being digested by the bile acids, or combining to produce gallstones. They are also fermented in the gut by bacteria which produce substances that are taken to the liver where they switch off the body's own cholesterol production.

Insoluble fibre is cereal bran from wheat, oats and other grains and it is best known as a remedy for constipation. Bran contains little water itself but it can absorb water and so bulk and soften faecal mass to help speedy evacuation from the body.

The fibre found in fruit called pectin dissolves in water but is resistant to digestive enzymes and it has a gelling and softening effect on stools.

Lignins are contained in the woody core of carrots and the tough outer leaves of cabbages and they are capable of binding with bile acids and drugs and removing them quickly from the body.

Although the presence of bran in food will help it to be digested more slowly and produce a steady rise in blood sugar rather than a sudden surge, such as happens with sugary low-fibre food, the gummy fibre in oats, beans and lentils is even more effective at this job.

Fibre will also slow the passage of food in the mouth and stomach helping to promote a feeling of satiety and because it keeps food in the stomach for longer it may result in better absorption of nutrients. Further down the gut it speeds things up and in the large intestine fibre is fermented by bacteria to produce gases which may result in flatulence associated with a high-fibre diet. It also produces short chain fatty acids which can be absorbed and used by the body.

The amount of fibre in the diet will also influence the type of bacteria that colonize the gut — the healthier combinations being found on a high-fibre diet, and a healthy bacterial flora can also help the liver and other organs in their work.

Fibre and Minerals

It has been claimed that the fibre present in wholegrains can prevent the body absorbing minerals such as iron, zinc and calcium that are present in these foods and vital for health. However studies on both animals and humans have had mixed results with some people (and some animals) showing no change in their mineral intake when extra dietary fibre is added to their food, some showing a slight decrease.

There have not been many long term studies but it is thought that the body will adapt to any adverse effect that fibre, and other closely associated substances such as phytate and tannin, might have. Some research on African men living in Gambia have shown that their high-fibre diet which is low in iron has led them to develop an improved efficiency for absorping any iron that is available in their diet.

Other studies have given a fibre supplement of cereals, fruit and nuts to people who usually eat a low-fibre diet to see if the fibre impaired their ability to absorb iron. During the short term of the trial there was no detrimental effect on iron status, and in fact the whole cereals, fruits and nuts provided more iron than their normal diet.

3.
HOW TO GET MORE FIBRE

Taking the easy way out and reaching for a packet of bran to sprinkle on food, or switching to a sugary bran breakfast cereal is not the best way to get more fibre. Adding bran to a diet based on refined foods such as white bread, cakes and pastries and high in meat and dairy produce is not the best way to go about it.

Changing to a pattern of eating that is overall more healthy is probably the best way to do it. Such a pattern is recommended in the NACNE report and gives good goals for both the long term and the short term. They are set out below. Putting all these recommendations into practice, along with giving up smoking and taking more exercise, will result in a much fitter and trimmer you and one who becomes happier because things will go better!

Recommendations of the NACNE Report

Food	Long term goals	Short term goals
Recommended daily intakes:		
Fibre (grams)	30	25
Sodium (milligrams)	3,600	4,300
Percentage of calories consumed:		
Fat	30	34
Saturated fat	10	15
Added sugar	10	12
Alcohol	4	5

For one thing fibre added as bran will not be effective in reducing blood cholesterol whereas eating both soluble and insoluble sources of fibre in wholefoods which are as near to their natural state as possible will do so. Bran may be an effective first aid measure but it is as unnatural as the ingredients of a refined diet in which the vitamins, minerals and fibre have been removed by food processing.

Overdoing the bran may also result in diarrhoea, irregular bowel habits and possibly small anal tears or fissures from over-large stools. The best way to increase fibre is to steadily switch to a natural, unprocessed diet which will provide a steady stream of energy and which comes complete with vitamins, minerals and fibre.

How Much to Aim For

The long term goals set by NACNE on page 25 will give you some idea, but trying to add up the amount of fibre you eat each day is no fun — unless you like measuring each mouthful against tables and charts and weighing everything you eat. It makes much more sense to apply the principles of a wholefood eating pattern and then you can happily forget about fibre and diet because it will take care of itself. A wholefood diet will provide the amount of fibre you need quite naturally without you having to think about it.

Generally the typical Western diet will provide between 15–25 grams of fibre a day which is about ½ to 1 ounce. This compares with 1½ to 2 ounces (40-60 grams) eaten in African populations. It doesn't sound like a lot but it makes all the difference. Most experts advise eating about 1½ ounces, or 30–35 grams a day and it is not recommended to exceed two ounces.

One long term study on a Dutch population of 1000 middle-aged men set the magic protective figure at 1½ ounces a day. Researchers studied the diets and medical histories of the men for 10 years and revealed that mortality was four times higher among low-fibre eaters.

To give you an idea about the fibre content of some common foods here is a list of the amount found in typical portions.

Wholemeal bread 2 slices	5 grams
1 apple	2 grams
Shredded Wheat, 2 biscuits	4.5 grams

1 banana	4.5 grams
Baked beans, 1 helping	5 grams
Muesli, 1 helping	6 grams

However, generally it is better to simply choose basic wholefoods and then replace the white varieties of most everyday foods with high-fibre varieties. For example:

Foods for Fibre in Wholefood Diet
Wholemeal bread, crispbreads
Wholemeal flour, soya flour and other whole grain flours
Oats, as porridge and oatcakes, in muesli and in baking
Wholemeal pastry, add some oats for extra soluble fibre
Brown rice and other whole grains such as millet, barley, cracked wheat, bulghur, etc
Pulses such as dried peas, beans and lentils — even baked beans
Fresh fruit — unpeeled
Fresh vegetables, unpeeled where possible, or cooked in their jackets like baked potatoes and sweet potatoes
Dried fruits such as apricots, prunes, dates, coconuts, raisins, sultanas, currants, peaches, pears
Nuts and seeds

Non-Fibre Foods in a Wholefood Diet
Free range eggs
Natural yogurt and strained yogurt in place of cream
No added sugar jams and marmalades
Fish, for essential fatty acids
Herb teas and mineral water, fruit juices and vegetable juices in place of some stimulant drinks such as tea and coffee and colas
Dry white wine or cider, in moderation, not more than two glasses a day
Cold pressed vegetable oils. Sunflower and safflower for salad dressings and corn oil or olive oil for cooking
Real cheese, choose mature flavours then you need only a little because cheese is a fatty food
Low-fat soft white cheeses and reduced-fat cheeses
Polyunsaturated margarines for spreading, or a little unsalted butter

Organically-grown Foods
Ask for organically-grown fruit and vegetables because they are produced without the use of artificial chemical fertilizers, sprays and pesticides etc.

Coeliacs
Coeliacs have an intolerance to gluten, the protein content of wheat, barley, rye and oats, so they cannot get their fibre from wholemeal bread or pasta or other grain sources. Brown rice, millet, whole corn, chickpeas and other beans and pulses, fresh fruit and vegetables, dried fruit and nuts with some soya bran or rice bran, if necessary.

Typical Day's High-Fibre Eating
Choose from the following suggestions

Breakfast
Wholemeal toast with little or no fat and some no-added sugar jams and marmalades or yeast extract

Home-made or bought no added sugar muesli

Other no added sugar or salt breakfast cereal such as Shredded Wheat, Cubs, Puffed Wheat, Kellogg's Nutrigrain range, Whole Earth granolas, Jordan's granola

Porridge made with rolled oats, or oatflakes or oatmeal with added oatbran and oatgerm if liked

Baked beans

Mushrooms on toast — sweated in stock, not fried

Scrambled egg — without added fat — or boiled or poached egg

Fresh fruit

Yogurt with dried fruit compote

Use skimmed milk on your cereal and in drinks

Fresh fruit or vegetable juice or mineral water to drink

Herb teas

Decaffeinated coffee or grain coffee

Lunch
Wholemeal sandwiches

Salad

Pitta bread and hummous

Open sandwiches
Pizza
Wholemeal pastie or pie
Pasta salad or bean salad
Savoury scones or rolls
Muesli
Wholemeal quiche

Evening meal
Soup with vegetables, pasta or pulses
Salads with raw or just blanched vegetables
Baked stuffed vegetables
Brown rice risotto, paella or pilau
Ethnic vegetarian dishes
Wholemeal pasta dishes
Wholemeal pies and quiches or pasties
Wholemeal pancakes with savoury stuffings

Desserts
Natural yogurt or fruit yogurt
Fresh fruit salads or platters, raw or cooked
Dried fruit compotes, fools, mousses, crumbles and tarts
Wholemeal pancakes
Grilled and stuffed fruits
Low-fat cheesecakes

Snacks
Wholemeal sandwiches
Nuts and seeds
Dried fruit
Fresh fruit
Oatcakes and other high-fibre savoury biscuits and crackers or
    crispbreads
Salads
Soups
Baked beans
Baked potatoes

4.

MENU SUGGESTIONS

Here are some menu suggestions that, taken together with the suggestions for breakfast and lunch will ensure a healthy intake of fibre between 33 and 50 grams a day. Most importantly they are completely natural foods, high in fibre and they do not rely on the unnatural addition of bran. Each ingredient is in its natural state.

The dishes are inter-changeable with others in the recipe section. Each recipe is marked with its fibre content per portion so it is possible for you to work out easily menus of your own choice that will add up to your daily fibre requirement.

Spring

Breakfast

Two wholemeal croissants   Two wholemeal croissants

Lunch

Four oatcakes with low-fat soft white cheese spread   Brown rice ring

Main Meal

Date and walnut salad   Fruit cocktail

★   ★

Tomato and olive pizza with Green bean and cashew salad	Broadbean minestrone with side salad of your choice
★	★
Hot fruit compote	Apricot and coconut crumble

Summer

Breakfast

Two breakfast buns	Two breakfast buns

Lunch

Pitta bread and salad	Niçoise pasta

Main Meal

Onion tart	Garden pea soup
★	★
Marrow hotpot	Avocado and Brazil pancakes
★	★
Apricot rice	Gooseberry cheesecake

Autumn

Breakfast

Fruity porridge	Fruity porridge

Lunch

Baked cabbage	Leek and potato quiche

Main Meal

Watercress soup	Melon salad
★	★
Moussaka with side salad	Topped vegetables with Parsnip cheese
★	★
Jack Horner crumble	Peach galette

Winter

Breakfast

Coconut muesli	Coconut muesli

Lunch

Lentil soup	Chilli baked potato

Main Meal

Persimmon cocktail	Celeriac soup
★	★
Dolmas	Groundnut stew with mangos and bananas
★	★
Prune jellies	Apricot gateau

Cooking Utensils

Aluminium saucepans have been the subject of suspicion for several years, mainly because they react with food. This can been seen when cooking acid foods, like fruit, in an aluminium pan. After cooking the pan is much shinier due to its reaction with the acid which may

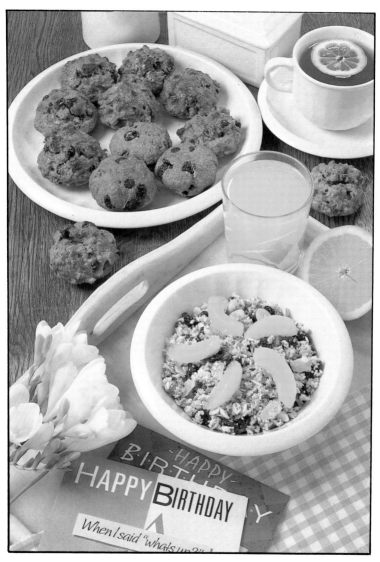

1. Breakfast: Breakfast Buns (page 38); Bran and Raisin Muffins (page 41) and Coconut Muesli (page 37).

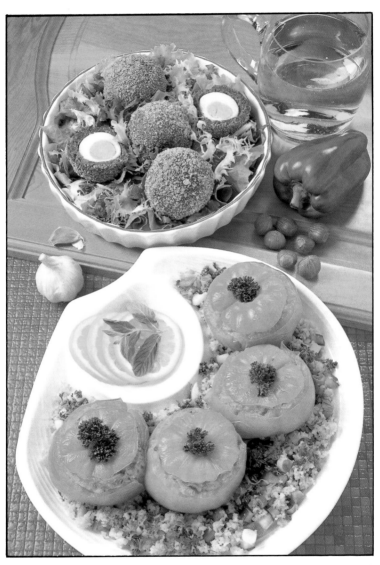

2. Light Meals I: Stuffed Tomatoes (page 105); Scotch Eggs (page 57); and Tabboulleh (page 58).

have made some aluminium come off into the food in minute amounts. These infinitesimal amounts may build up in the body over the years. Aluminium is not an 'essential nutrient' for the body and it may even be harmful. For this reason it is best to choose stainless steel pans that do not react with food. Glassware, ceramic material and cast iron or enamelled cookware can also be used.

Meat and 'Complete' Protein

This cookbook has not consciously set out to exclude meat but because meat is devoid of fibre and high in saturated fats it does not make a useful contribution to a book that aims to outline practical ways to healthier eating.

Many of the vegetable dishes may be served with meat and they will usefully boost the fibre content of such a meal.

Fish is preferred to meat because it is an excellent source of protein and its fat is unsaturated. It also provides essential fatty acids that are beneficial to health.

The recipes in this book provide protein from vegetable sources because these are also sources of fibre. Vegetable proteins are not the 'complete' proteins that meat, fish and dairy proteins are; they contain only a few of the essential building blocks needed by the body to make its own protein. However by mixing proteins from vegetable sources 'complete' proteins can be formed by the body.

To achieve complete proteins make sure the meal contains one of the following three combinations:

● grains (cereal, pasta, rice etc.) with legumes (beans, peas or lentils);
● grains and milk products;
● seeds (sesame, sunflower, pumpkin) and legumes.

PART 2
THE RECIPES

5.

BREAKFASTS

COCONUT MUESLI *Illustrated in colour*
Serves 4.
5g fibre/250 calories per portion.

Imperial (Metric)	American
4 tablespoonsful rolled oats	⅓ cupful rolled oats
2 tablespoonsful millet flakes	2 tablespoonsful millet flakes
1 tablespoonful sunflower seeds	1 tablespoonful sunflower seeds
1 tablespoonful raisins	1 tablespoonful raisins
1 tablespoonful flaked almonds	1 tablespoonful slivered almonds
1 tablespoonful ground coconut	1 tablespoonful ground coconut
1 tablespoonful wheatgerm	1 tablespoonful wheatgerm

1. Mix all ingredients together very thoroughly to ensure fair shares of the nuts and raisins!

2. Place portions of muesli in breakfast bowls and soak overnight, in either fruit juice such as apple juice, or mineral water. Natural yogurt or cultured buttermilk may also be used.

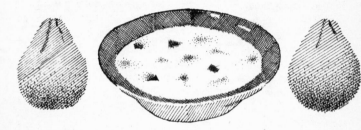

SIMPLE MUESLI *Illustrated in colour*
Serves 2.
3g fibre/300 calories per portion.

Imperial (Metric)
6 tablespoonsful rolled oats
1 tablespoonful raisins
1 tablespoonful sunflower seeds
Apple juice or mineral water
1 tablespoonful hazelnuts
1 eating apple

American
½ cupful rolled oats
1 tablespoonful raisins
1 tablespoonful sunflower seeds
Apple juice or mineral water
1 tablespoonful hazelnuts
1 eating apple

1. Mix together the oats, raisins and sunflower seeds. Soak overnight in apple juice or water in the fridge.

2. Next morning chop the hazelnuts and grate the cored but unpeeled apple. Stir these into the muesli.

3. Add more juice or water or, if preferred, top with natural yogurt before serving.

BREAKFAST BUNS
Makes about 16.
3g fibre/110 calories each.

Imperial (Metric)
6 oz (150g) wholemeal flour
2 teaspoonsful baking powder
2 oz (50g) bran
2 oz (50g) polyunsaturated
    margarine
2 tablespoonsful clear honey
5 fl oz (150ml) apple juice
4 oz (100g) raisins
4 oz (100g) walnuts, chopped
1 cooking apple, grated

American
1½ cupsful wholewheat flour
2 teaspoonsful baking soda
½ cupful bran
¼ cupful polyunsaturated margarine
2 tablespoonsful clear honey
⅔ cupful apple juice
⅔ cupful raisins
¾ cupful chopped English walnuts
1 cooking apple, grated

1. Sieve the flour and baking powder into a bowl. Stir in the bran.

2. Place the margarine, honey and apple juice in a saucepan over gentle heat and melt.

3. Stir the raisins, walnuts and apple into the dry ingredients.

4. Pour over the melted ingredients and mix thoroughly. The mixture will be quite moist.

5. Place 1 tablespoonful of mixture into lightly oiled bun tins or paper bun cases.

6. Bake at 375°F/190°C (Gas Mark 5) for 25 minutes.

FRUITY PORRIDGE
Serves 4.
4½g fibre/240 calories per portion.

Imperial (Metric)	American
6 oz (150g) rolled oats	1½ cupsful rolled oats
2 oz (50g) wheatgerm	½ cupful wheatgerm
2 oz (50g) raisins	⅓ cupful raisins
Water	Water
2 eating apples	2 eating apples

1. Place the oats, wheatgerm and raisins in a saucepan.

2. Add water and place over low heat. Bring to simmering point, stirring continuously to prevent sticking. The amount of water needed will depend on the absorbency of the oats and the texture at which porridge is preferred. Between ½ pint (¼ litre)/1⅓ cupsful and ¾ pint (400ml)/2 cupsful will probably be enough.

3. Core, but do not peel the apples, and grate them into the porridge just before serving.

WHOLEMEAL CROISSANTS

Makes 24.
2½g fibre/70 calories each.

Imperial (Metric)	American
1 oz (25g) fresh yeast, or	2½ tablespoonsful fresh yeast, or
½ oz (12g) dried yeast	1 tablespoonful dried yeast
1 vitamin C tablet	1 vitamin C tablet
⅓ pint (200ml) warm water	1 cupful warm water
⅓ pint (200ml) evaporated milk	1 cupful evaporated milk
2 oz (50g) unsalted butter, melted	¼ cupful unsalted butter, melted
1½ lb (675g) wholemeal flour	6 cupsful wholewheat flour
1 teaspoonful sea salt (optional)	1 teaspoonful sea salt (optional)
6 oz (150g) unsalted butter	¾ cupful unsalted butter
Milk to glaze	Milk to glaze

1. Crumble the yeast and crushed vitamin C tablet into the warm water.

2. Add the evaporated milk and stir well.

3. Melt the smaller amount of butter in saucepan. Remove from heat.

4. Sieve the flour and salt (if used) into a bowl.

5. Rub the larger amount of butter into the flour until it resembles breadcrumbs.

6. Make a well in centre of the flour and pour in the yeast mixture and melted butter and mix thoroughly.

7. Turn onto a lightly floured surface and knead for 5 minutes. Return to bowl, cover and leave to rest for 10 minutes.

8. Turn ⅓ dough onto a lightly floured surface and roll into a circle with dough about ¼ in. (7mm) thick.

9. Using a sharp knife cut the dough into eight segments. Working from the outside, roll each triangular segment into the middle to form a croissant roll. Bend into a crescent moon shape and place on lightly oiled baking tray. Cover and leave to double in size.

10. Repeat with other ⅔ dough, or leave covered in fridge and use when fresh croissants are required. Dough will keep for up to four days.

11. Glaze with milk and bake at 350°F/180°C (Gas Mark 4) for 30 minutes. Best eaten same day.

BRAN AND RAISIN MUFFINS *Illustrated in colour*
Makes 8
5 grams fibre/150 calories each

Imperial (Metric)	American
⅛ pint (75ml) skimmed milk	⅓ cupful skimmed milk
2 oz (50g) soft vegetable margarine	¼ cupful soft vegetable margarine
1 oz (25g) molasses	1 tablespoonful molasses
2 oz (50g) malt or barley extract	¼ cupful malt extract
6 oz (150g) wholemeal flour	1½ cupfuls wholewheat flour
1 teaspoonful baking powder	1 teaspoonful baking powder
2 oz (50g) bran	½ cupful bran
2 oz (50g) raisins	¼ cupful raisins

1. Place the milk, margarine, molasses and malt extract in a saucepan and heat until all are melted together. Stir well.

2. Sift the flour and baking powder into a bowl and add the bran from the sieve, plus the extra bran.

3. Stir in the raisins and then pour on the liquid and mix well.

4. Place in lightly-oiled muffin or bun tin and bake in a pre-set oven at 375°F/190°C (Gas Mark 5) for 20–25 minutes until risen and golden brown. Nice hot or cold.

6.

STARTERS, SOUPS AND SALADS

FRUIT COCKTAIL
Serves 4.
3g fibre/65 calories per glass.

Imperial (Metric)	American
1 grapefruit	1 grapefruit
1 lemon	1 lemon
1 orange	1 orange
1 lime	1 lime
1 small fresh pineapple, or tin pineapple in its own juice	1 small fresh pineapple, or can pineapple in own juice
Perrier or similar naturally sparkling mineral water	Perrier or similar naturally sparkling mineral water

1. Cut pith and peel from the citrus fruits and roughly chop. Remove pips. Place fruit in a liquidizer.

2. Cut skin from the pineapple and remove central core if very woody. Chop and add to liquidizer.

3. Liquidize fruits and place in a large jug. Cover.

4. Make the juice only just before serving to minimize vitamin loss. To cool, stir in ice cubes and add sparkling water to taste.

FELAFEL

Makes 14
1.6g fibre/60 calories each

Imperial (Metric)	American
1 red pepper, diced	1 red pepper, diced
1 clove garlic, crushed	1 clove garlic, crushed
1 onion, diced	1 onion, diced
1 tablespoonful vegetable oil	1 tablespoonful vegetable oil
14 oz (400g) tin chickpeas	2 cupfuls cooked garbanzo beans
1 tablespoonful freshly chopped parsley	1 tablespoonful freshly chopped parsley
Freshly ground black pepper	Freshly ground black pepper
1 teaspoon ground coriander	1 teaspoon ground coriander
2 free range hard-boiled eggs	2 free range hard-boiled eggs

1. Place the pepper, garlic and onion in a saucepan with the oil and cook until soft.

2. Remove from the heat and liquidize with the chickpeas to a thick purée.

3. Place in a bowl and stir in the parsley and seasoning.

4. Finely chop the eggs and add to the mixture then mould into egg-shaped balls (done more easily with wet hands) and place in the fridge until required.

MELON SALAD *Illustrated in colour*
Serves 4.
5g fibre/100 calories per portion.

Imperial (Metric)	American
1 large canteloupe melon	1 large canteloupe melon
1 papaya	1 papaya
½ lb (¼ kilo) strawberries	2 cupsful strawberries
2 oranges	2 oranges

1. Cut the melon in half. Remove seeds and reserve juice.

2. Using a Parisienne cutter (melon baller) scoop balls from the flesh.

3. Halve the papaya and remove seeds. Slice thinly.

4. Arrange the melon balls, papaya and slices of strawberry on serving plates and pour over the freshly squeezed juice of 2 oranges.

5. Chill for 30 minutes before serving.

HUMMOUS
Dip for 6–8 people
2-1.5 grams fibre/1050 calories in total

Imperial (Metric)	American
14 oz (400g) tin chickpeas	2 cupfuls cooked garbanzo beans
5 oz (150g) tahini	⅔ cupful tahini
Juice of 3 lemons	Juice of 3 lemons
2 cloves garlic, crushed	2 cloves garlic, crushed
Freshly ground black pepper	Freshly ground black pepper
Freshly chopped parsley, as garnish	Freshly chopped parsley, as garnish

1. Place all the ingredients except the parsley in a food processor and blend to a smooth purée.

2. Place in a bowl and rough the top with a fork, sprinkle with parsley and serve.

You can add a spoonful or two of olive oil to the mixture or trickle over the top before serving, if liked.

2. Peel and crush the garlic and add to the *puréed* chick peas (garbanzos). Stir in lemon juice, seasoning and tahini to taste.

3. Place the hummus in a serving dish and garnish with parsley.

SUMMER OMELETTE
Serves 4.
8g fibre/290 calories per portion.

Imperial (Metric)	American
1 lb (½ kilo) new potatoes	1 pound new potatoes
½ lb (¼ kilo) new carrots	8 ounces new carrots
½ lb (¼ kilo) peas	1⅓ cupsful peas
6 free-range eggs	6 free-range eggs
Sea salt	Sea salt
Freshly ground black pepper	Freshly ground black pepper
1 tablespoonful freshly chopped basil	1 tablespoonful freshly chopped basil
1 oz (25g) unsalted butter or corn oil	2½ tablespoonsful unsalted butter or corn oil

1. Scrub, but do not peel, the potatoes and carrots. Steam or boil until just cooked. Drain.

2. Cook the peas until just tender. Drain.

3. Dice the potatoes and carrots and mix with the peas.

4. Whisk eggs well and season. Stir in basil.

5. Place fat in a large omelette pan and allow butter to melt and foam, but not brown.

6. Pour in the omelette mixture. As it begins to set, lift edges with a palette knife and allow unset mixture to run underneath and set.

7. Place the vegetables in the centre of the omelette and cook for a minute or so. Fold the omelette in half to envelop the vegetables and carefully lift onto a serving plate. Cut into 4 and eat immediately. Alternatively make smaller omelettes.

GARDEN PEA SOUP *Illustrated in colour*
Serves 4.
11g fibre/140 calories per portion.

Imperial (Metric)
2 lb (1 kilo) garden-fresh peas
1 bunch spring onions
1½ pints (¾ litre) vegetable stock or
  water
1 tablespoonful single cream
1 tablespoonful chopped chives
Sea salt
Freshly ground black pepper

American
2 pounds garden-fresh peas
1 bunch scallions
3¾ cupsful vegetable stock or water
1 tablespoonful light cream
1 tablespoonful chopped chives
Sea salt
Freshly ground black pepper

1. Shell the peas and place in a large saucepan.

2. Chop the spring onions (scallions) and add to the peas.

3. Add boiling stock or water. Simmer for about 20 minutes or until peas are cooked. Remove from heat.

4. When cool, sieve or liquidize.

5. Add cream, chives and seasoning to taste.

6. Good either hot or cold.

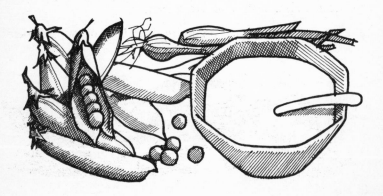

SUMMER VEGETABLE SOUP

Serves 4.
6½g fibre/220 calories per portion.

Imperial (Metric)	American
8 baby carrots, washed	8 baby carrots
½ lb (¼ kilo) peas, shelled	8 ounces peas, shelled
8 baby new potatoes, scrubbed	8 baby new potatoes, scrubbed
6 oz (150g) tender young French or runner beans	6 ounces tender young snap or green beans
1 bunch spring onions	1 bunch scallions
2 small courgettes, sliced	2 small zucchini, sliced
1 oz (25g) unsalted butter or vegetable oil	2½ tablespoonsful unsalted butter or vegetable oil
1½ pints (¾ litre) vegetable stock or water	3¾ cupsful vegetable stock or water
Sea salt	Sea salt
Freshly ground black pepper	Freshly ground black pepper
Natural yogurt	Natural yogurt

1. Place the roughly chopped vegetables in a saucepan with butter or oil. Cover and cook gently for 5 minutes.

2. Add stock or water and simmer for 15 minutes or until the vegetables are just cooked.

3. Season to taste and spoon equal amounts of each vegetable into each serving dish. Pour stock over.

4. Swirl a teaspoonful of yogurt into each bowl of soup just before serving.

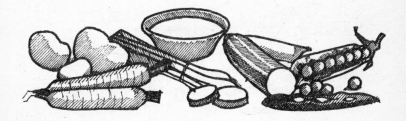

CELERIAC SOUP

Serves 4.
7g fibre/30 calories per portion.

Imperial (Metric)
½ lb (¼ kilo) onion, chopped
4 oz (100g) carrot, chopped
1 lb (½ kilo) celeriac, chopped
1 pint (½ litre) vegetable stock
Sea salt
Freshly ground black pepper

American
1¼ cupful chopped onion
⅔ cupful chopped carrot
2⅔ cupful chopped celeriac
2½ cupful vegetable stock
Sea salt
Freshly ground black pepper

1. Place the onion and carrot in a heavy-based saucepan and *sauté* for five minutes.

2. Add the celeriac and stock. Cover and simmer for 20 minutes.

3. Liquidize the mixture and return to saucepan.

4. Season to taste and re-heat.

5. Serve with home-made wholemeal bread for a satisfying meal and extra fibre.

WATERCRESS SOUP

Serves 4.
3½g fibre/90 calories per portion.

Imperial (Metric)
2 bunches watercress
¾ lb (350g) potatoes
1 onion
2 pints (1 litre) vegetable stock
Bouquet garni
Sea salt
Freshly ground black pepper

American
2 bunches watercress
12 ounces potatoes
1 onion
5 cupful vegetable stock
Bouquet garni
Sea salt
Freshly ground black pepper

1. Wash the watercress well in plenty of cold water. Discard any yellowing leaves.

2. Scrub the potatoes and roughly chop.

3. Peel and dice the onion.

4. Place all the ingredients in a large saucepan with well-fitting lid and bring to boil.

5. Lower heat and simmer for 15 minutes or until the vegetables are cooked.

6. Remove from heat and allow to cool slightly. Remove the bouquet garni before liquidizing.

7. Chill before serving.

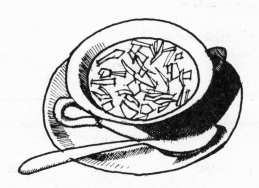

LENTIL SOUP

Serves 4.
6½g fibre/200 calories per portion.

Imperial (Metric)	American
½ lb (¼ kilo) lentils	1 cupful lentils
1 teaspoonful freshly grated ginger root	1 teaspoonful freshly grated root ginger
½ teaspoonful ground turmeric	½ teaspoonful ground turmeric
1 teaspoonful ground coriander	1 teaspoonful ground coriander
20 peppercorns and 20 cloves tied in muslin bag	20 peppercorns and 20 cloves tied in muslin bag
2 pints (1 litre) water	5 cupsful water
1 oz (25g) unsalted butter	2½ tablespoonsful unsalted butter
1 teaspoonful cumin seeds	1 teaspoonful cumin seeds
1 dried chilli, diced	1 dried chilli, diced
2 ripe tomatoes, diced	2 ripe tomatoes, diced

1. Pick over the lentils, removing all grit and stones and wash well.

2. Place the lentils, ginger, turmeric, coriander and muslin bag in a saucepan with water.

3. Bring to boil, lower heat and simmer for 30 minutes.

4. Melt the butter in a separate pan and add cumin seeds and chilli. *Sauté* for 2 minutes being careful not to burn the butter.

5. Add the diced tomatoes and cook for further 2 minutes.

6. Remove bag of cloves from soup. Liquidize for smooth soup and return to pan.

7. Stir the tomato mixture into the soup and serve immediately.

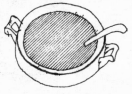

WINTER SALAD

Serves 6
2 grams fibre/40 calories per portion

Imperial (Metric)	American
1 lemon	1 lemon
½ small white cabbage	½ small white cabbage
2 large carrots	2 large carrots
3 sticks celery	3 stalks celery
1 red eating apple	1 red eating apple
1 small onion	1 small onion
1½ oz (40g) sultanas	¼ cupful golden seedless raisins
3 tablespoonsful cold pressed oil mayonnaise	3 tablespoonsful cold pressed oil mayonnaise
Freshly ground black pepper	Freshly ground black pepper

1. Squeeze the juice from the lemon.

2. Grate the cabbage and carrots by hand or in a food processor.

3. Finely dice the celery and eating apple and toss all the vegetables together in a bowl with the lemon juice.

4. Finely dice the onion and stir in, together with the sultanas, the mayonnaise and the pepper.

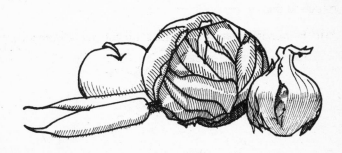

DATE AND WALNUT SALAD

Serves 4.
5½g fibre/240 calories per portion.

Imperial (Metric)	American
6 sticks celery, sliced	6 stalks celery, sliced
2 eating apples, diced but not peeled	2 eating apples, diced but not peeled
Juice of ½ lemon	Juice of ½ lemon
4 oz (100g) walnuts, chopped	¾ cupful English walnuts, chopped
4 oz (100g) dates, chopped	1 cupful dates, chopped
½ lb (¼ kilo) cottage cheese	1 cupful cottage cheese

1. Toss the prepared celery and apple in lemon juice.

2. Add the nuts and dates to the apple mixture.

3. Stir in the cheese, and mix thoroughly.

KOHLRABI SALAD

Serves 4.
3g fibre/80 calories per portion.

Imperial (Metric)	American
1 lb (½ kilo) kohlrabi	1 pound kohlrabi
½ lb (¼ kilo) carrots	8 ounces carrots
6 oz (150g) onion	6 ounces onion
2 sticks celery	2 sticks celery
Salad dressing (page 51)	Salad dressing (page 51)

1. Scrub and grate the kohlrabi and carrot.

2. Peel and finely dice the onion and slice the celery.

3. Mix together the salad dressing ingredients and pour over the prepared vegetables. Toss before serving.

GREEN BEAN AND CASHEW SALAD

Serves 4.
3½g fibre/220 calories per portion.

Imperial (Metric)
1 lb (½ kilo) French or dwarf English
  green beans
5 oz (125g) cashew nuts
1 tablespoonful cold-pressed
  safflower mayonnaise

American
1 pound snap beans
1 cupful cashew nuts
1 tablespoonful cold-pressed
  safflower mayonnaise

1. Top and tail the beans and wash well.

2. Place the beans in a small amount of boiling water, cover and cook for 5 minutes. Drain and refresh with cold water.

3. Chop the cashews, or leave whole if preferred.

4. Toss the beans and cashews in mayonnaise and serve warm or cold.

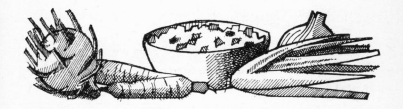

7.

LIGHT MEALS

MILLET BURGERS
Makes 4.
3½g fibre/240 calories per portion.

Imperial (Metric)	American
4 oz (100g) millet	½ cupful millet
6 oz (150g) onion, diced	1 cupful diced onions
2 oz (50g) mature English cheddar cheese, grated	½ cupful grated hard cheese
1 tablespoonful chopped parsley	1 tablespoonful chopped parsley
1 tablespoonful stoneground mustard	1 tablespoonful stoneground mustard
2 free-range eggs, beaten	2 free-range eggs, beaten
4 oz (100g) wholemeal breadcrumbs	1 cupful wholewheat breadcrumbs

1. Place the millet in a saucepan of boiling water. Cover and cook until soft, about 20 minutes. Drain.

2. Place the millet, onion, cheese, parsley, mustard, ⅔ of the egg and half the breadcrumbs in a bowl and bind together into burger or large sausage shapes.

3. Roll the burgers in the beaten egg and coat in remaining breadcrumbs.

4. Lightly fry in a small amount of vegetable oil or bake in moderate oven on lightly oiled baking tray until golden brown. Turn once during cooking.

LENTIL PATTIES
Makes 16
0.5 grams fibre/45 calories each

Imperial (Metric)	American
4 oz (100g) whole continental lentils	¾ cupful lentils
6 oz (175g) cottage cheese	1¼ cupsful cottage cheese
1 teaspoonful fenugreek seeds, ground	1 teaspoonful fenugreek seeds, ground
1 teaspoonful garam masala	1 teaspoonful garam masala
2 oz (50g) maize flour	½ cupful maize flour
Vegetable oil to fry	Vegetable oil to fry

1. Pick over the lentils and remove any grit or stones, then wash and place in a saucepan with plenty of water to cover. Boil for 30 minutes and drain if necessary, then place in a food processor.

2. Add the cheese and the spices, blending to a soft consistency. Stir in the flour to thicken. Form into patties and then fry in a little oil. Pat with absorbent kitchen paper to remove excess oil after frying.

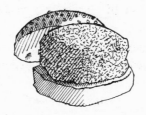

WALNUT BURGERS

Makes 4.
6g fibre/400 calories per burger.

Imperial (Metric)	American
4 oz (100g) ground walnuts	1 cupful ground walnuts
4 oz (100g) ground hazelnuts	1 cupful ground hazelnuts
4 oz (100g) fresh wholemeal breadcrumbs	2 cupsful fresh wholewheat breadcrumbs
1 onion, peeled and diced	1 onion, peeled and diced
Clove garlic, crushed	Clove garlic, crushed
1 level tablespoonful freshly chopped parsley	1 level tablespoonful freshly chopped parsley
1 teaspoonful freshly chopped thyme	1 teaspoonful freshly chopped thyme
2 free-range eggs	2 free-range eggs
Water to mix	Water to mix
2 oz (50g) sesame seeds	⅓ cupful sesame seeds

1. Place the nuts, breadcrumbs, onion, garlic and herbs in a mixing bowl and mix thoroughly.

2. Beat one egg with two tablespoonsful of water and stir into the nut mixture. Add more water, if necessary, to bind the mixture.

3. Shape into four burgers.

4. Beat the second egg and use to dip burgers in before rolling in sesame seeds.

5. Grill for 20 minutes, turning once. Alternatively bake on a lightly oiled baking tray for 20 minutes, turning once, at 375°F/190°C (Gas Mark 5).

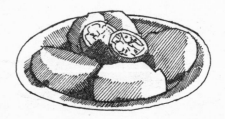

TABBOULLEH *Illustrated in colour*
Serves 4–6
1.5-1 grams fibre/100-65 calories per serving

Imperial (Metric)
4 oz (100g) burghul
½ cucumber, diced
1 green pepper, finely diced
4 spring onions, diced
2 tablespoonful freshly chopped
  parsley
1 tablespoonful freshly chopped mint
Juice of ½ lemon

American
½ cupful burghul
½ cucumber, diced
1 green pepper, finely diced
4 scallions, diced
2 tablespoonsful freshly chopped
  parsley
1 tablespoonful freshly chopped mint
Juice of ½ lemon

1. Boil the burghul in twice its volume of water for about 10 minutes.

2. Drain, if necessary, and squeeze out excess moisture, then place in a bowl and stir in the rest of the ingredients.

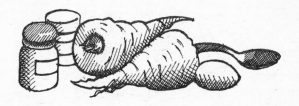

SCOTCH EGG *Illustrated in colour*
Makes 4
3 grams fibre/250 calories each

Imperial (Metric)	American
4 free range hard-boiled eggs	4 free range hard-boiled eggs
1 free range egg, beaten	1 free range egg, beaten
4 oz (100g) ground hazelnuts	1 cupful ground hazelnuts
2 tablespoonsful no added sugar tomato ketchup	2 tablespoonsful no added sugar tomato ketchup
2 teaspoonsful chopped sage	2 teaspoonsful chopped sage
1 finely chopped onion	1 finely chopped onion
1 tablespoonful sesame seed oil	1 tablespoonful sesame seed oil
2 oz (50g) wholemeal breadcrumbs	1 cupful wholewheat breadcrumbs
Freshly ground black pepper	Freshly ground black pepper

1. Lightly oil a baking tray and set the oven to 375°F/190°C (Gas Mark 5).

2. Shell the eggs and place on one side with the beaten egg.

3. Mix together the rest of the ingredients to form a thick paste.

4. Dip the eggs in the beaten egg and mould the paste around them.

5. Place the eggs on the baking tray and bake for 20 minutes, turning once.

6. Allow to cool before serving.

These eggs are baked rather than deep fried to reduce their calorie content. They taste just as good!

SAVOURY SWEET POTATOES

Serves 4.
5g fibre/290 calories per portion.

Imperial (Metric)	American
2 large sweet potatoes	2 large sweet potatoes
½ lb (¼ kilo) low-fat curd cheese	1 cupful low-fat curd cheese
2 free-range egg yolks	2 free-range egg yolks
4 shallots, finely diced	4 shallots, finely diced
1 tablespoonful chopped chives	1 tablespoonful chopped chives
Sea salt	Sea salt
Freshly ground black pepper	Freshly ground black pepper

1. Scrub the potatoes and bake, unpeeled, at 400°F/200°C (Gas Mark 6) for 1 hour. Remove from oven.

2. Cut the potatoes in half and scoop out most of the flesh, leaving enough to hold the potato skin in shape.

3. Beat together the potato flesh, cheese, egg yolks, shallots and seasoning.

4. Pile mixture back into shells and return to oven to heat through.

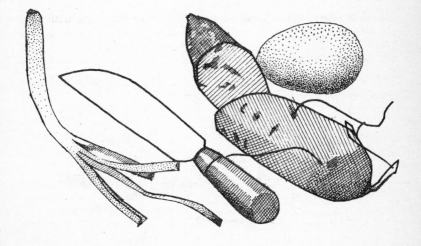

STILTON YAMS

Serves 4.
4½g fibre/260 calories per portion.

Imperial (Metric)	American
1½ lb (¾ kilo) yam or sweet potato	1½ pounds yam or sweet potato
¼ pint (150ml) skimmed milk	⅔ cupful skimmed milk
Freshly ground black pepper	Freshly ground black pepper
Sea salt	Sea salt
3 oz (75g) watercress, finely chopped	1½ cupsful watercress, finely chopped
4 oz (100g) white Stilton or Caerphilly cheese	1 cupful Stilton or hard cheese of choice

1. Scrub the yams and slice into 1 in. (25mm) thick rounds.

2. Place in a large, heavy-based saucepan with well-fitting lid and pour milk over them.

3. Season generously and place lid on pan. Simmer for 10 minutes until slices are just cooked. Drain.

4. Place the slices in a lightly oiled gratin dish and cover with watercress.

5. Pare thin slices of cheese, using a cheese plane and place on top of the watercress.

6. Grill until cheese is just melting.

7. Serve with home-made chutney.

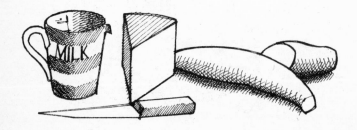

CHILLI BAKED POTATOES

Serves 4.
19g fibre/360 calories per portion.

Imperial (Metric)	American
4 large potatoes, scrubbed and baked in their skins	4 large potatoes, scrubbed and baked in their skins
½ lb (¼ kilo) red kidney beans	1⅓ cupsful red kidney beans
6 oz (150g) onion, peeled and diced	1 cupful diced onion
2 fresh chillies, diced	2 fresh chillies, diced
1 teaspoonful vegetable oil	1 teaspoonful vegetable oil
1 small tin tomatoes	1 small tin tomatoes

1. Soak the beans overnight. Drain and boil in plenty of water for 45 minutes, or until soft.

2. While the beans are cooking bake the potatoes.

3. *Sauté* the onion in oil with the chillies.

4. Add the tomatoes and beans and simmer together for a further 15 minutes.

5. Remove the potatoes from oven. Cut a deep cross in tops, squeeze open and pour bean mixture over them.

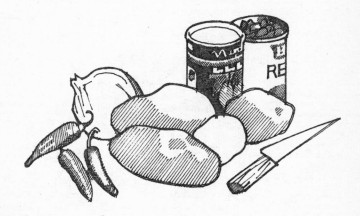

CABBAGE BAKED POTATOES

Serves 4.
8g fibre/240 calories per potato.

Imperial (Metric)
4 large potatoes, scrubbed and
 baked in their skins
½ lb (¼ kilo) white cabbage,
 shredded
½ lb (¼ kilo) cooking apple, cored
 and grated
4 oz (100g) sultanas
Sea salt
Freshly ground black pepper

American
4 large potatoes, scrubbed and
 baked in their skins
2 cupsful shredded white cabbage
1⅓ cupsful cooking apple, cored and
 grated
⅔ cupful golden seedless raisins
Sea salt
Freshly ground black pepper

1. While the potatoes are baking prepare the vegetables and place
    in a large heavy-based saucepan with well-fitting lid.

2. Add a little water and cover. Cook gently for 30 minutes.

3. After 10 minutes add sultanas (golden seedless raisins). Season
    to taste.

4. Remove the cooked potatoes from oven. Halve, and spoon cabbage
    mixture over.

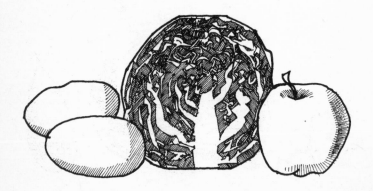

BROAD BEAN MINESTRONE

Serves 4.
6g fibre/140 calories per portion.

Imperial (Metric)	American
2 lb (1 kilo) broad beans	5⅓ cupful Windsor beans
2 tablespoonsful olive oil	2 tablespoonsful olive oil
4 oz (100g) onion, diced	⅔ cupful diced onion
4 oz (100g) carrot, diced	⅔ cupful diced carrot
1 stick celery, chopped	1 stalk celery, chopped
2 pints (1 litre) vegetable stock	5 cupful vegetable stock
Pinch sea salt	Pinch sea salt
½ lb (¼ kilo) wholemeal spaghetti broken into small pieces	2 cupful wholewheat spaghetti broken into small pieces
Parmesan cheese (optional)	Parmesan cheese (optional)

1. Shell the beans.

2. Heat oil in a saucepan and add the onion, carrot and celery. Cover and *sauté* for 5 minutes.

3. Add the beans and stock and bring to boil. Lower heat to simmering point for 20 minutes.

4. Stir in the spaghetti and simmer for further 10 minutes or until spaghetti is *al dente* (cooked, but still firm when bitten).

5. Serve at once, with a bowl of cheese for those who want it.

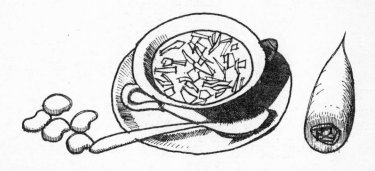

BEAN AND PASTA SALAD

Serves 4
7.5 grams fibre/300 calories per portion

Imperial (Metric)
4 oz (100g) wholemeal macaroni or other pasta shapes
6 oz (150g) broad beans shelled weight
14 oz (400g) tin cooked chickpeas
Juice 1 orange
Freshly ground black pepper
Freshly chopped parsley or chives
1 teaspoonful meux mustard
3 tablespoonsful olive oil

American
2 cupsful wholewheat pasta shapes
1 cupful shelled Windsor beans
2 cupsful cooked garbanzo beans
Juice 1 orange
Freshly ground black pepper
Freshly chopped parsley or chives
1 teaspoonful meux mustard
3 tablespoonsful olive oil

1. Boil the pasta in plenty of water until cooked but *al dente* that is still offering some resistance when bitten. Drain and run under cold water to stop the cooking.

2. Boil the beans and when cooked drain and add to the pasta.

3. Drain the tin of chickpeas and add to the beans and pasta.

4. Place the orange juice, pepper, herbs and mustard in a clean screwtop jar with the oil and shake vigorously to combine into a salad dressing. Pour over the warm ingredients and serve at once or when cold.

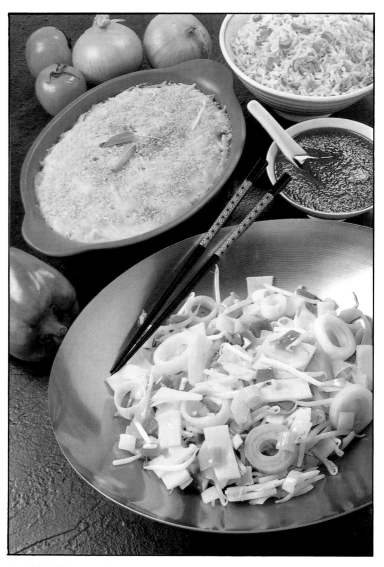

3. Light Meals II: Stir-Fry Vegetables (page 86); Parsnip and Tomato Bake (page 96).

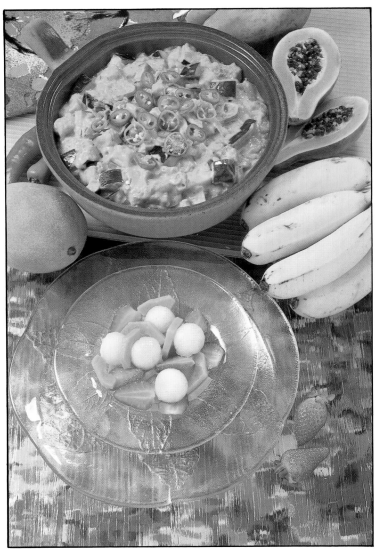

4. Main Meal Menu I: Melon Salad (page 44); Groundnut Stew and Mangoes (page 73).

8. Bake at 400°F/200°C (Gas Mark 6) for 35-40 minutes, until topping is golden brown and set.

BROAD BEAN TAGLIATELLI
Serves 4.
10g fibre/270 calories per portion.

Imperial (Metric)	American
3 fl oz (85ml) olive oil	1/3 cupful olive oil
2 cloves garlic, crushed	2 cloves garlic, crushed
1 dried chilli, chopped	1 dried chilli, chopped
1 tablespoonful freshly chopped parsley	1 tablespoonful freshly chopped parsley
1/2 pint (1/4 litre) vegetable stock	1 1/3 cupful vegetable stock
3/4 lb (350g) broad beans, shelled	2 cupsful shelled Windsor beans
4 oz (100g) garden peas, shelled	2/3 cupful shelled garden peas
1/2 lb (1/4 kilo) wholemeal tagliatelli	1 1/2 cupsful wholewheat tagliatelli

1. Place the olive oil, garlic, chilli and parsley in a saucepan. Cover and *sauté* for 5 minutes.

2. Add the stock, beans and peas. Cover and simmer for 20 minutes.

3. Boil the tagliatelli in plenty of salted (optional) water for 12 minutes, or until *al dente* (that is, still firm to the teeth when bitten, but just cooked). Drain.

4. Place the tagliatelli on serving dish and pour bean sauce over it.

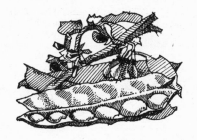

LASAGNE
Serves 4.
12g fibre/300 calories per portion.

Imperial (Metric)	American
½ lb (¼ kilo) wholemeal lasagne	8 ounces wholewheat lasagne
1 oz (25g) wholemeal flour	¼ cupful wholewheat flour
1 oz (25g) unsalted butter or polyunsaturated margarine	2½ tablespoonsful unsalted butter, or polyunsaturated margarine
¼ pint (150ml) vegetable stock	⅔ cupful vegetable stock
½ lb (¼ kilo) spinach, cooked and chopped	1 cupful spinach, cooked and chopped
Freshly ground nutmeg, to taste	Freshly ground nutmeg, to taste
Freshly ground black pepper	Freshly ground black pepper
½ lb (¼ kilo) onion, diced	1⅓ cupsful diced onion
1 clove garlic, crushed	1 clove garlic, crushed
1 lb (½ kilo) tomatoes, chopped	1 pound tomatoes, chopped
1 medium red pepper, diced	1 medium red pepper, diced
4 oz (100g) carrots, diced	⅔ cupful diced carrots
4 oz (100g) cashew nuts, chopped	¾ cupful chopped cashew nuts
1 tablespoonful basil	1 tablespoonful basil
1 tablespoonful oregano	1 tablespoonful oregano
Freshly ground black pepper	Freshly ground black pepper

1. Place the lasagne in saucepan with plenty of boiling water and cook for about 12 minutes, or until *al dente* (cooked, but still firm to the teeth when bitten). Drain and separate sheets.

2. Place the flour and butter in saucepan and cook together, stirring continuously over a low heat.

3. Gradually add the vegetable stock, stirring all the time as the sauce thickens.

4. Stir in the spinach and seasoning.

5. In another saucepan place the onion and garlic. Cover and *sauté* for 5 minutes.

6. Add the tomatoes, pepper and carrots. Cover and cook for a further 10 minutes. Stir in the nuts, herbs and seasoning to taste.

7. Lightly oil an ovenproof dish and place a layer of the tomato mixture in the base. Cover with a layer of lasagne.

8. On top of the lasagne place a layer of the spinach mixture and top with more lasagne. Repeat once more, ending with spinach mixture.

9. Bake at 375°F/190°C (Gas Mark 5) for 30 minutes. Serve with a green salad.

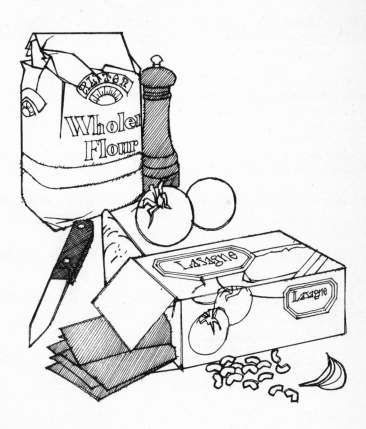

SPAGHETTI BUTTER BEANS

Serves 4.
18g fibre/270 calories per portion.

Imperial (Metric)	American
½ lb (¼ kilo) butter beans	1⅓ cupsful wax beans
½ lb (¼ kilo) onion, diced	1⅓ cupsful diced onion
2 cloves garlic, crushed	2 cloves garlic, crushed
1 tablespoonful olive oil	1 tablespoonful olive oil
1 lb (½ kilo) tomatoes, roughly chopped	1 pound tomatoes, roughly chopped
2 sticks celery, finely sliced	2 stalks celery, finely sliced
¼ pint (150ml) vegetable stock	⅔ cupful vegetable stock
Bouquet garni	Bouquet garni
2 tablespoonsful freshly chopped parsley	2 tablespoonsful freshly chopped parsley
½ lb (¼ kilo) wholemeal spaghetti	8 ounces wholewheat spaghetti
1 large carrot, grated	1 large carrot, grated

1. Boil the beans in plenty of boiling water until almost cooked. Drain.

2. Place the onion and garlic in a heavy-based saucepan with oil. Cover with a well-fitting lid and *sauté* for 5 minutes.

3. Add the tomatoes, beans, celery, stock, bouquet garni and parsley. Cover and simmer for 20 minutes.

4. Boil the spaghetti in plenty of water for about 12 minutes until *al dente* (firm to the teeth when bitten, but just cooked). Drain.

5. Place spaghetti in a serving dish. Stir the grated carrot into the bean mixture and pour over spaghetti.

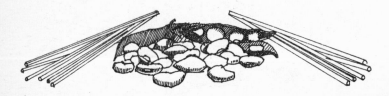

FENNEL PASTA

Serves 4.
12g fibre/350 calories per portion.

Imperial (Metric)	American
2 large fennel bulbs, diced	2 large fennel bulbs, diced
½ lb (¼ kilo) onion, diced	1⅓ cupful onion, diced
1 large red pepper, diced	1 large red pepper, diced
1 tablespoonful olive oil	1 tablespoonful olive oil
¼ pint (150ml) vegetable stock	⅔ cupful vegetable stock
4 oz (100g) raisins	⅔ cupful raisins
4 oz (100g) flaked almonds	1 cupful slivered almonds
Sea salt	Sea salt
Freshly ground black pepper	Freshly ground black pepper
½ lb (¼ kilo) wholemeal pasta shells	4 cupful wholewheat pasta shells

1. Place the fennel, onion and pepper in a saucepan with the oil. Cover with a well-fitting lid and *sauté* over low heat for 10 minutes.

2. Add stock, raisins, almonds and seasoning. Cover and simmer for 20 minutes.

3. While this is cooking boil the pasta in a large saucepan with plenty of boiling water for about 12 minutes, or until *al dente* (that is, still firm when bitten, but just cooked). Drain.

4. Place the pasta in a serving dish and cover with fennel sauce. Toss well and serve.

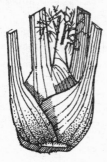

RED BEANS AND PASTA

Serves 4.
10g fibre/260 calories per portion.

Imperial (Metric)	American
3 oz (75g) red kidney beans	½ cupful red kidney beans
3 oz (75g) blackeye beans	½ cupful blackeye beans
6 oz (150g) wholemeal pasta shells	3 cupsful wholewheat pasta shells
1 small can soyaprotein frankfurters	1 small can soyaprotein frankfurters

Dressing:

Imperial (Metric)	American
2 tablespoonsful olive oil	2 tablespoonsful olive oil
1 tablespoonful wine vinegar	1 tablespoonful wine vinegar
1 teaspoonful ready mixed stoneground mustard	1 teaspoonful ready mixed stoneground mustard
Freshly ground black pepper	Freshly ground black pepper

1. Place the beans in a saucepan of boiling water and boil fiercely for at least 10 minutes. Continue cooking until soft — about 45 minutes if the beans are fresh. Drain and cool.

2. Place the pasta shells in boiling water and cook for about 12 minutes until *al dente* (still slightly firm when bitten, but just cooked). Drain and cool.

3. If the frankfurters are not ready to eat, cook according to manufacturer's instructions and allow to cool.

4. Combine the dressing ingredients in a screwtop jar and shake well.

5. Place all salad ingredients in serving bowl and toss in dressing.

8.

MAIN MEALS

ADUKI ROAST
Serves 4.
6g fibre/390 calories per portion.

Imperial (Metric)	American
1 lb (½ kilo) cooked aduki beans	2 cupsful cooked aduki beans
¼ pint (150ml) tomato sauce (page 104)	⅔ cupful tomato sauce (page 104)
4 oz (100g) walnuts, ground	1 cupful ground English walnuts
4 oz (100g) peanuts, ground	1 cupful ground peanuts
3 oz (75g) rolled oats	¾ cupful rolled oats
4 oz (100g) wholemeal breadcrumbs	2 cupsful wholewheat breadcrumbs
½ lb (¼ kilo) onion, finely diced	1⅓ cupsful finely diced onion
4 oz (100g) carrot, finely grated	⅔ cupful finely grated carrot
1 tablespoonful freshly chopped parsley	1 tablespoonful freshly chopped parsley
2 free-range eggs	2 free-range eggs

1. Place the cooked beans in a liquidizer with a few tablespoonsful of tomato sauce, and *purée*.

2. Add the rest of the ingredients and blend together. For a rougher texture mix *puréed* beans in a bowl with the other ingredients. Use chopped nuts rather than ground nuts, if preferred.

3. Turn the mixture into a lightly oiled loaf tin and bake at 375°F/190°C (Gas Mark 5) for 1 hour.

PAELLA

Serves 4
9 grams fibre/250 calories per serving

Imperial (Metric)	American
6 oz (150g) whole continental lentils	1 cupful whole continental lentils
6 oz (150g) brown rice	¾ cupful brown rice
1 clove garlic, crushed	1 clove garlic, crushed
1 large onion, diced	1 large onion, diced
1 red pepper, diced	1 red pepper, diced
1 green pepper, diced	1 green pepper, diced
2 tablespoonsful olive oil	2 tablespoonsful olive oil
½ teaspoonful turmeric	½ teaspoonful turmeric
6 oz (150g) French beans, sliced	1 cupful French beans, sliced
2 courgettes, sliced	2 zucchini, sliced
1 pint (600ml) vegetable stock	2½ cupsful vegetable stock
4 tomatoes, halved	4 tomatoes, halved
4 oz (100g) peas	⅔ cupful peas
Freshly ground black pepper	Freshly ground black pepper
Pinch paprika	Pinch paprika

1. Wash and pick over the lentils and rice and boil them for 15 minutes.

2. In the paella pan fry the garlic, onion and peppers in the oil until slightly softened.

3. Add the drained rice and lentils and stir in thoroughly with the turmeric to colour the mixture.

4. Add the beans and courgettes and pour over the stock. Simmer gently for about 30 minutes, topping up with liquid as required, until the rice is cooked.

5. Add the tomatoes and peas about 15 minutes before the end of cooking, arranging the tomatoes, cut sides uppermost, around the edge of the pan. Season with pepper and paprika to taste. The best paellas are made without stirring or disturbing the rice during cooking — so resist the temptation!

EILEEN'S GROUNDNUT STEW AND MANGOES

Serves 4. *Illustrated in colour*
13g fibre/470 calories per portion.

Imperial (Metric)

½ lb (¼ kilo) onion, diced
1 fresh chilli, finely chopped
½ teaspoonful fresh ginger, grated
1 teaspoonful vegetable oil
1 lb (½ kilo) tomatoes (canned or fresh)
½ lb (¼ kilo) crunchy peanut butter
1 lb (½ kilo) aubergines
4 oz (100g) okra
2 mangoes
2 bananas

American

1⅓ cupsful onion, diced
1 fresh chilli, finely chopped
½ teaspoonful fresh ginger, grated
1 teaspoonful vegetable oil
1 pound tomatoes (canned or fresh)
2 cupsful crunchy peanut butter
1 pound eggplants
4 ounces okra
2 mangoes
2 bananas

1. Place the onion, chilli and ginger in a heavy-based saucepan. Add oil, cover with a well-fitting lid and *sauté* gently for five minutes.

2. Stir in the tomatoes and break them up with back of spoon.

3. Add the peanut butter and simmer for 20 minutes.

4. Meanwhile wash and dice the unpeeled aubergines (eggplants) and steam or boil for 20 minutes.

5. Wash and remove stems from the okra. Steam or boil for ten minutes.

6. Stir the aubergines (eggplants) and okra into the peanut mixture and continue cooking for 5 minutes.

7. Peel and slice the mangoes and bananas and mix together.

8. Serve the groundnut stew and offer the bananas and mangoes separately. Best served with brown rice.

PECAN ROAST

Serves 4.
8g fibre/600 calories per portion.

Imperial (Metric)
10 oz (300g) pecan nuts
½ lb (¼ kilo) wholemeal breadcrumbs
½ lb (¼ kilo) onion, finely diced
½ lb (¼ kilo) carrot, finely grated
Juice of ½ lemon
Sea salt
Freshly ground black pepper
2 free-range eggs

American
2 cupsful pecan nuts
4 cupsful wholewheat breadcrumbs
1⅓ cupsful finely diced onion
1⅓ cupsful finely grated carrot
1 tablespoonful freshly chopped sage
Juice of ½ lemon
Sea salt
Freshly ground black pepper
2 free-range eggs

1. Grind or chop the pecan nuts, depending on preferred texture of the roast.

2. Stir in the breadcrumbs, onion, carrot, sage, lemon juice and seasoning.

3. Add the beaten eggs to bind the mixture. If more liquid is needed use a little vegetable stock.

4. Turn the mixture into a lightly oiled loaf tin and bake at 375°F/190°C (Gas Mark 5) for 45 minutes.

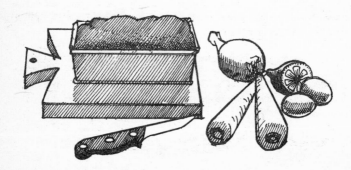

WHOLEMEAL PANCAKES
Makes 10.
2½g fibre/75 calories per pancake.

Imperial (Metric)
4 oz (100g) wholemeal flour
Pinch sea salt (optional)
1 free-range egg, beaten
½ pint (¼ litre) skimmed milk, or
 ¼ pint (150ml) milk and ¼ pint
 (150ml) water

American
1 cupful wholewheat flour
Pinch sea salt (optional)
1 free-range egg, beaten
1⅓ cupful skimmed milk or
 ⅔ cupful milk and ⅔ cupful water

1. Sieve the flour and salt into a mixing bowl.

2. Make a well in centre and add the egg.

3. Stir flour into the liquid working from the centre towards the sides of bowl. Keep the paste smooth and avoid lumps by working slowly.

4. Gradually add milk to mixture, and beat well when all liquid is worked in.

5. To ensure light pancakes use a heavy-based omelette pan. Heat a smear of oil in the pan before adding mixture and pour only enough batter in to cover the base of the pan when the mixture is thinly spread.

6. Turn the pancakes once after loosening with flexible palette knife.

Note: To make a complete meal out of pancakes, see the following recipes for exciting fillings.

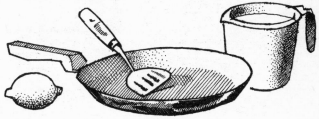

SPINACH PANCAKES
Makes 10.
6g fibre/145 calories per pancake.

Imperial (Metric)	American
½ lb (¼ kilo) frozen spinach, or 1 lb (½ kilo) fresh spinach	1 cupful frozen spinach, or 1 pound fresh spinach
1 tablespoonful wholemeal flour	1 tablespoonful wholewheat flour
1 tablespoonful unsalted butter or polyunsaturated margarine	1 tablespoonful unsalted butter or polyunsaturated margarine
¼ pint (150ml) skimmed milk	⅔ cupful skimmed milk
Grated fresh nutmeg	Grated fresh nutmeg
Pinch sea salt	Pinch sea salt
Freshly ground black pepper	Freshly ground black pepper
3 oz (75g) mature English Cheddar cheese grated	¾ cupful hard cheese of choice, grated

1. Make the pancakes (page 75).

2. Wash fresh spinach in plenty of cold water to remove all dirt and grit. Slice with a sharp knife.

3. Place in a large saucepan and cover with a well-fitting lid. Cook for about 5 minutes, turning once or twice. There is no need to add more water to cook the spinach in. If using frozen spinach, drain well after defrosting, then heat gently.

4. Add the flour and butter or margarine to the spinach and stir in well.

5. Gradually add milk, stirring continuously, to thicken mixture.

6. Season to taste and divide the mixture into equal amounts for each pancake. Roll up the pancakes and place in an ovenproof dish.

7. Sprinkle cheese over the pancakes and bake at 350°F/180°C (Gas Mark 4) for 20 minutes.

BROCCOLI AND CASHEW PANCAKES
Makes 10.
4g fibre/100 calories per pancake.

Imperial (Metric)
½ lb (¼ kilo) broccoli spears
2 oz (50g) cashew nuts, finely
   chopped
1 tablespoonful freshly chopped
   parsley
1 oz (25g) ground coconut
1 free-range egg, beaten
¼ pint (150ml) natural yogurt
Sea salt
Freshly ground black pepper

American
8 ounces broccoli spears
½ cupful cashew nuts, finely
   chopped
1 tablespoonful freshly chopped
   parsley
⅓ cupful ground coconut
1 free-range egg, beaten
⅔ cupful natural yogurt
Sea salt
Freshly ground black pepper

1. Make the pancakes (page 75).

2. Steam or boil the broccoli for 4 minutes in minimum amount of water.

3. Mix the nuts, parsley, coconut, natural yogurt and egg together in a bowl.

4. Place some broccoli on each pancake and spoon the nut mixture over. Roll the pancakes up.

5. Place the pancakes in a lightly oiled ovenproof dish. Cover and bake at 375°F/190°C (Gas Mark 5) for 25-30 minutes.

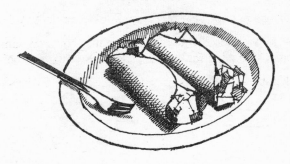

AVOCADO AND BRAZIL PANCAKES *Illustrated in colour*

Makes 10.

· 4g fibre/270 calories per pancake.

Imperial (Metric)
2 ripe avocados
½ lemon
2 oz (50g) Brazil nuts, finely
  chopped
2 tablespoonsful freshly chopped
  parsley
4 oz (100g) tomatoes, chopped
1 oz (25g) wholemeal breadcrumbs
2 tablespoonsful tomato sauce
  (page 104)

American
2 ripe avocados
½ lemon
½ cupful Brazil nuts, finely chopped
2 tablespoonsful freshly chopped
  parsley
4 ounces tomatoes, chopped
½ cupful wholewheat breadcrumbs
2 tablespoonsful tomato sauce
  (page 104)

1. Peel and slice the avocados. Dress with lemon juice to prevent browning.

2. Mix together the nuts, parsley, tomatoes and breadcrumbs and stir in the avocado slices.

3. Add tomato sauce to bind and place a tablespoonful of mixture on each pancake. Roll up.

4. Place the pancakes in an ovenproof dish and cover. Bake at 400°F/200°C (Gas Mark 6) for 15 minutes.

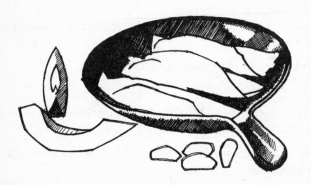

TOPPED VEGETABLES

Serves 4.
9g fibre/280 calories per portion.

Imperial (Metric)	American
½ lb (¼ kilo) swede, diced	1⅓ cupsful diced rutabaga
½ lb (¼ kilo) carrots, sliced	1⅓ cupsful sliced carrots
½ lb (¼ kilo) shelled peas	1⅓ cupsful shelled peas
2 tablespoonsful chopped parsley	2 tablespoonsful chopped parsley
½ pint (¼ litre) vegetable stock	1⅓ cupsful vegetable stock

Topping:

Imperial (Metric)	American
1 oz (25g) unsalted butter or polyunsaturated margarine	2½ tablespoonsful unsalted butter or polyunsaturated margarine
2 oz (50g) mashed potato	¼ cupful mashed potato
2 oz (50g) mature English Cheddar cheese, grated	½ cupful hard cheese of choice, grated
2 oz (50g) oatmeal	½ cupful oatmeal
4 oz (100g) wholemeal flour	1 cupful wholewheat flour
Sea salt	Sea salt
Freshly ground black pepper	Freshly ground black pepper
1 tablespoonful skimmed milk	1 tablespoonful skimmed milk

1. Steam or boil the swede and carrots for 5 minutes. Blanch the peas for 1 minute.

2. Mix the vegetables with the parsley and stock and place in an ovenproof dish.

3. Cream the fat and potato together.

4. Mix the cheese, oatmeal, flour and seasoning and add to the potato.

5. Add enough water to form a soft dough and roll out. Carefully lift it onto the vegetables to form a pastry-style crust.

6. Glaze with milk and bake at 400°F/200°C (Gas Mark 6) for 30 minutes.

MOUSSAKA

Serves 4.
10g fibre/670 calories per portion.

Imperial (Metric)	American
1 lb (½ kilo) aubergines	1 pound eggplants
1 tablespoonful olive oil	1 tablespoonful olive oil
¾ lb (350g) onion, diced	2 cupsful diced onion
1 clove garlic, crushed	1 clove garlic, crushed
1 lb (½ kilo) tomatoes, chopped	1 pound tomatoes, chopped
2 tablespoonsful freshly chopped parsley	2 tablespoonsful freshly chopped parsley
½ lb (¼ kilo) crunchy peanut butter	2 cupsful crunchy peanut butter
¼ pint (150ml) tomato sauce (page 104)	⅔ cupful tomato sauce (page 104)
Sea salt	Sea salt
Freshly ground black pepper	Freshly ground black pepper

Topping:

Imperial (Metric)	American
1 oz (25g) polyunsaturated margarine	2½ tablespoonsful polyunsaturated margarine
1 oz (25g) wholemeal flour	¼ cupful wholewheat flour
½ pint (¼ litre) skimmed milk	1⅓ cupsful skimmed milk
2 oz (50g) rolled oats	½ cupful rolled oats
Pinch sea salt (optional)	Pinch sea salt (optional)
Freshly ground black pepper	Freshly ground black pepper
3 oz (75g) mature English Cheddar	¾ cupful hard cheese of choice
2 free-range eggs, separated	2 free-range eggs, separated

1. Wash and slice the aubergines (eggplants). Blanch in boiling water for 3 minutes. Drain.

2. Heat half the oil in large non-stick frying pan (skillet) and *sauté* the aubergines (eggplants) for 10 minutes, turning once.

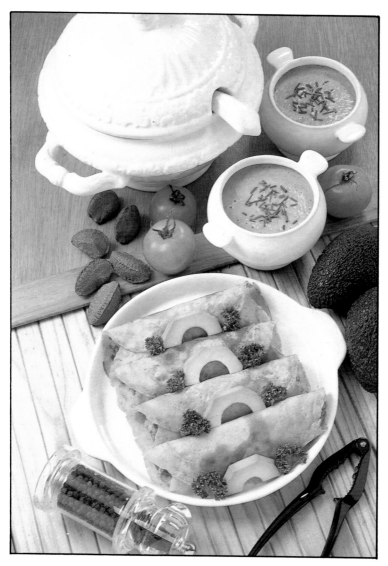

5. Main Meal II: Garden Pea Soup (page 46); Avocado and Brazil Pancakes (page 78).

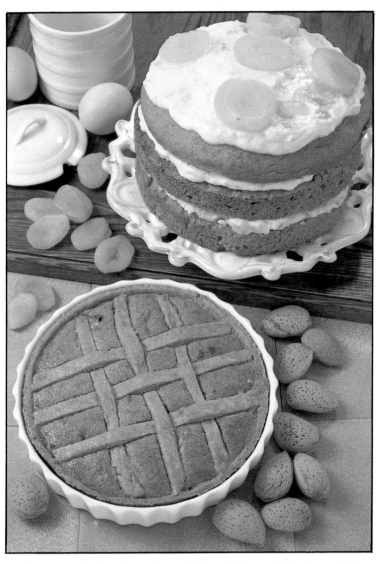

6.   Desserts: Apricot Gateau (page 126) and Bakewell Tart (page 120).

3. In another pan *sauté* the onions and garlic for 5 minutes.

4. Add the tomatoes to the onions, plus the parsley and stir in the peanut butter and tomato sauce. Heat through.

5. Place a layer of aubergines (eggplants) in an ovenproof dish. Top with a layer of tomato mixture and repeat until the mixture is used up. Set aside.

6. To make the topping, place the fat and flour in a heavy-based saucepan over low heat and make a *roux* (thick paste) by stirring continuously.

7. Gradually add milk, still stirring to prevent lumps forming.

8. When all the liquid has been added remove from heat and stir in the oats and seasoning.

9. Add the cheese and egg yolks.

10. Whisk egg whites to firm peaks and quickly fold into the mixture.

11. Pour immediately over vegetable mixture and bake at 375°F/190°C (Gas Mark 5) for 40 minutes or until topping is risen and golden.

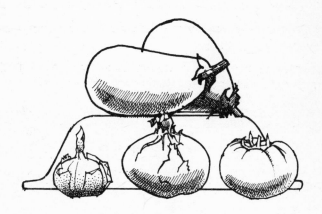

TOMATO AND OLIVE PIZZA
Serves 4.
8½g fibre/250 calories per portion.

Dough:

Imperial (Metric)	American
½ lb (¼ kilo) wholemeal flour	2 cupsful wholewheat flour
¼ oz (7g) fresh yeast	2 teaspoonsful fresh yeast
¼ pint (150ml) warm water	⅔ cupful warm water
1 teaspoonful vegetable oil	1 teaspoonful vegetable oil
½ vitamin C tablet, crushed	½ vitamin C tablet, crushed

Topping:

Imperial (Metric)	American
14 oz (400g) tin tomatoes	1 medium can tomatoes
½ lb (¼ kilo) onion, diced	1⅓ cupsful diced onion
1 clove garlic, crushed	1 clove garlic, crushed
1 large red pepper, deseeded and diced	1 large red pepper, deseeded and diced
4 oz (100g) carrots, grated	⅔ cupful grated carrot
2 tablespoonsful freshly chopped parsley	2 tablespoonsful freshly chopped parsley
2 oz (50g) black olives	½ cupful black olives
Freshly ground black pepper	Freshly ground black pepper
4 oz (100g) Mozzarella cheese	½ cupful Mozzarella cheese

1. Sieve the flour and salt into a bowl.

2. Crumble the yeast into warm water and stir in the oil and vitamin C tablet.

3. Pour the water onto the flour and mix to a dough.

4. Turn onto a floured surface and knead for 5 minutes.

5. Return the dough to the bowl and cover. Leave to rest for 10 minutes.

6. Place the tomatoes in a saucepan over low heat and break up with a fork. Add the onion, garlic, pepper and carrot and cook for 10 minutes, or until nicely thickened.

7. Stir in the parsley, remove from heat and season to taste.

8. Return the pizza dough to the floured surface and roll out. Place on a large pizza dish, or make 4 smaller rounds and place on a lightly oiled baking tray.

9. Spread the tomato mixture on top of dough and arrange the olives on the mixture.

10. Slice the Mozzarella thinly and place on top of the pizza. Bake at 400°F/200°C (Gas Mark 6) for 25 minutes.

Alternative toppings: A small can of anchovy fillets can be added to the tomato paste. Sliced mushrooms can be added to the mixture, or as decoration. Tuna fish goes well with pizza toppings.

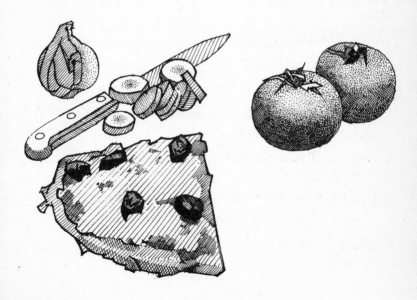

PEASE PUDDING

Serves 4.
6g fibre/210 calories per portion.

Imperial (Metric)	American
½ lb (¼ kilo) yellow split peas	1 cupful yellow split peas
4 oz (100g) onion, diced	⅔ cupful diced onion
1 bay leaf	1 bay leaf
1 pint (½ litre) vegetable stock	2½ cupsful vegetable stock
1 teaspoonful freshly chopped sage	1 teaspoonful freshly chopped sage
1 oz (25g) polyunsaturated margarine	2½ tablespoonsful polyunsaturated margarine
1 free-range egg	1 free-range egg

1. Soak the peas overnight in hot water. Drain.

2. Place the peas in a saucepan with the onion, bay leaf, stock and sage. Cover. Bring to boil and simmer for 1½ hours until peas are cooked. Watch the pot to ensure it does not boil dry and burn. Top up with water if necessary.

3. When the peas are cooked, cool and *purée* in a liquidizer with the seasoning, margarine and egg.

4. Turn the mixture into a lightly oiled pudding basin and cover with greaseproof paper and a pudding cloth or aluminium foil. Secure and steam for 45 minutes.

5. Turn out and serve hot with vegetables or cold with salad.

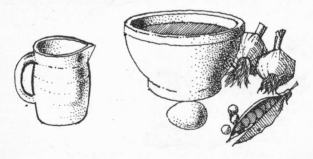

BAKED NUT CABBAGE

Serves 4.
7g fibre/280 calories per portion.

Imperial (Metric)
1½ lb (⅔ kilo) green cabbage
Freshly ground black pepper
2 oz (50g) unsalted butter or
 polyunsaturated margarine
¼ pint (150ml) vegetable stock
Pinch ground mace
2 oz (50g) salted peanuts
2 oz (50g) mature English Cheddar
 cheese

American
1½ pounds green cabbage
Freshly ground black pepper
¼ cupful unsalted butter or
 polyunsaturated margarine
⅔ cupful vegetable stock
Pinch ground mace
⅓ cupful salted peanuts
½ cupful hard cheese of choice

1. Using a sharp knife shred the cabbage finely and wash well.

2. Heat a little water in large saucepan. When boiling, drop in the cabbage and season with pepper. Simmer for 5 minutes. Drain, reserving liquid.

3. In another saucepan melt the butter and flour, stirring well to make a *roux* (thick paste). Gradually stir in the vegetable stock and enough water from the cabbage to make a creamy sauce. Season with mace.

4. Lightly oil an ovenproof dish and place a layer of cabbage in the bottom.

5. Cover with a little sauce and sprinkle some nuts and cheese on top of the sauce. Repeat the process, ending with a cheese layer.

6. Bake at 400°F/200°C (Gas Mark 6) for 15 minutes.

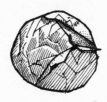

STIR-FRY VEGETABLES *Illustrated in colour*

Serves 4.
5½g fibre/270 calories per portion.

Imperial (Metric)	American
½ lb (¼ kilo) brown rice	1 cupful brown rice
2 leeks	2 leeks
1 large onion	1 large onion
1 tablespoonful sesame oil	1 tablespoonful sesame oil
1 green pepper	1 green pepper
10 oz (300g) tin bamboo shoots	1 medium can bamboo shoots
4 oz (100g) beansprouts	2 cupsful beansprouts

1. Wash the rice and place in a saucepan with 2½ times its volume of boiling water. Cover and simmer for 40 minutes.

2. Scrub and slice the leeks.

3. Peel and dice the onion and place, with the leek, in a wok, or frying pan (skillet) with the oil. *Sauté* for 3 minutes.

4. Wash and de-seed the pepper. Dice and add to wok.

5. Drain the can of bamboo shoots. Slice thinly and add to wok.

6. Wash the beansprouts and, just before serving, stir into vegetables. Allow to heat through and serve hot with the rice and Sweet and Sour Sauce if liked (page 88).

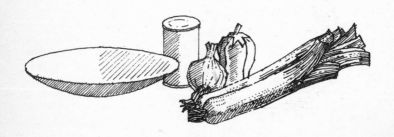

STIR-FRY VEGETABLES AND BEANS

Serves 4.
5g fibre/360 calories per portion.

Imperial (Metric)	**American**
½ lb (¼ kilo) brown rice	1 cupful brown rice
1 tablespoonful sesame oil	1 tablespoonful sesame oil
Large onion, diced	Large onion, diced
1 clove garlic, crushed	1 clove garlic, crushed
2 carrots, cut into matchsticks	2 carrots, cut into matchsticks
1 large head broccoli, divided into florets	1 large head broccoli, divided into florets
1 red pepper, de-seeded and cut into strips	1 red pepper, de-seeded and cut into strips
½ lb (¼ kilo) cooked blackeye beans	1 cupful cooked blackeye beans

1. Wash the rice and put it in a saucepan with 2½ times its volume of water. Cover and bring to boil. Cook for 40 minutes.

2. Heat the oil in a wok and *sauté* the onion and garlic for 5 minutes.

3. Add the other vegetables, stirring all the time to prevent sticking and help even cooking.

4. Just before serving stir in the beans and heat through.

5. Serve with Sweet and Sour Sauce (page 88).

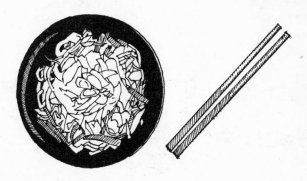

SWEET AND SOUR SAUCE

0g fibre/196 calories total.

Imperial (Metric)	American
1 orange	1 orange
2 tablespoonsful red wine vinegar	2 tablespoonsful red wine vinegar
1 tablespoonful Demerara sugar	1 tablespoonful Demerara sugar
1 dessertspoonful tomato *purée*	2 teaspoonsful tomato paste
2 tablespoonsful water	2 tablespoonsful water
2 tablespoonsful soya sauce	2 tablespoonsful soy sauce

1. Cut the orange in half and squeeze juice.

2. Place juice with all the other ingredients in saucepan and heat gently until all ingredients are thoroughly combined.

3. Pour over Stir-fry Vegetables (pages 86 and 87).

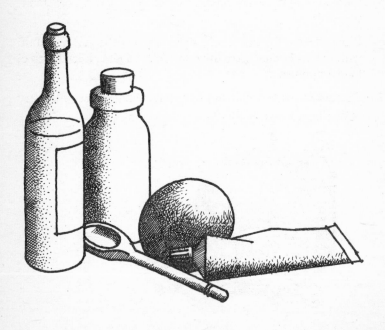

WHOLEMEAL PASTRY FLAN CASE
3½g fibre/260 calories.

Imperial (Metric)
6 oz (150g) wholemeal flour
3 oz (75g) polyunsaturated
  margarine
1 free-range egg yolk, beaten
Water to mix

American
1½ cupsful wholewheat flour
⅓ cupful polyunsaturated margarine
1 free-range egg yolk, beaten
Water to mix

1. Sieve the flour into a mixing bowl.

2. Rub in fat until the mixture resembles breadcrumbs in texture.

3. Make a well in the centre and stir in the yolk and water to make a soft dough.

4. Turn onto a floured surface and roll out.

5. Carefully fold in half and lift into a lightly oiled flan ring or ceramic flan dish.

6. Place a layer of greaseproof paper on top of the pastry and fill with baking beans. Bake blind at 400°F/200°C (Gas Mark 6) for 10 minutes.

7. Remove from oven and lift out the paper and beans. The pastry case is now ready for filling.

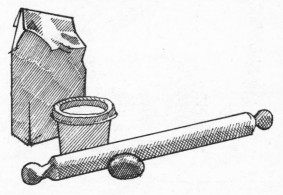

ONION TART

Serves 4.
4½g fibre/359 calories per portion.

Imperial (Metric)
10 oz (300g) onion, diced
4 oz (100g) quark, or similar low-fat,
   soft white cheese
¼ pint (150ml) natural yogurt
2 free-range eggs
Sea salt (optional)
Freshly ground black pepper
Pinch of ground mace
Baked blind pastry case (page 89)

American
1⅔ cupsful diced onion
½ cupful quark, or similar low-fat,
   soft white cheese
⅔ cupful natural yogurt
2 free-range eggs
Sea salt (optional)
Freshly ground black pepper
Pinch of ground mace
Baked blind pastry case (page 89)

1. Place the onions in a frying pan (skillet) smeared with a little vegetable oil, and *sauté* for 5 minutes.

2. Beat together the cheese, yogurt, eggs and seasoning.

3. Put the onions onto absorbent paper to drain off any excess fat, and turn them into the prepared pastry case.

4. Pour the yogurt mixture on top and bake at 400°F/200°C (Gas Mark 6) for 35 minutes or until golden brown and set.

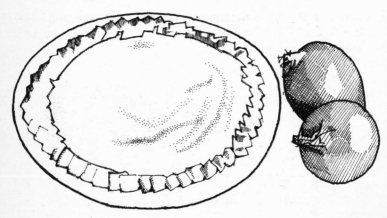

LEEK AND POTATO QUICHE

Serves 4.
7g fibre/390 calories per portion.

Imperial (Metric)	American
¾ lb (350g) potatoes	12 ounces potatoes
½ lb (¼ kilo) leeks	8 ounces leeks
¼ pint (150ml) natural yogurt	⅔ cupful natural yogurt
1 free-range egg, separated	1 free-range egg, separated
Sea salt	Sea salt
Freshly ground black pepper	Freshly ground black pepper
Baked blind pastry case (page 89)	Baked blind pastry case (page 89)

1. Scrub the potatoes and dice, but do not peel.

2. Slice the leeks and wash well.

3. Place the potatoes and leeks in a saucepan with a smear of vegetable oil. Cover and cook for 5 minutes.

4. Beat together the yogurt, egg yolk and seasoning.

5. Place the leeks and potatoes on absorbent kitchen paper to remove any excess oil, then turn into the prepared pastry case.

6. Whisk the egg white to stiff peaks and fold into the yogurt mixture.

7. Pour over the top of the vegetables in the pastry case and bake at 375°F/190°C (Gas Mark 5) for 35 minutes or until golden brown and firm to the touch.

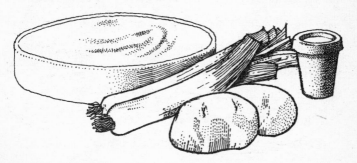

CHILLI BEANS

Serves 4.
20g fibre/260 calories per portion.

Imperial (Metric)	American
10 oz (300g) kidney beans, soaked overnight	1²/₃ cupsful kidney beans, soaked overnight
1 tablespoonful vegetable oil	1 tablespoonful vegetable oil
½ lb (¼ kilo) green pepper, de-seeded and diced	8 ounces green pepper, de-seeded and diced
4 oz (100g) onion, diced	²/₃ cupful diced onion
2 cloves garlic, crushed	2 cloves garlic, crushed
4 fresh chillis, de-seeded and finely diced	4 fresh chillis, de-seeded and finely diced
14 oz (400g) tin tomatoes	1 medium can tomatoes
¼ pint (150ml) vegetable stock	²/₃ cupful vegetable stock
1½ teaspoonsful ground cumin	1½ teaspoonsful ground cumin
1 teaspoonful oregano	1 teaspoonful oregano
Sea salt (optional)	Sea salt (optional)
½ lb (¼ kilo) broccoli, divided into florets	8 ounces broccoli, divided into florets

1. Drain the soaked beans and put them in a saucepan of boiling water. Cook for about 40 minutes, or until soft.

2. Heat the oil in a heavy-based saucepan.

3. Add the pepper, onion, garlic and chillies and *sauté*, covered, for 10 minutes.

4. Add the tomatoes and break them up with a wooden spoon.

5. Add the vegetable stock and cook for a further 10 minutes.

6. Stir in cumin, oregano and salt.

7. Add the broccoli florets and cook for further 5 minutes.

8. Stir in the cooked beans. Heat through.

9. Serve with brown rice for a complete protein meal.

CRACKED WHEAT PASTIES
Makes 6–8
5.5–4g fibre/225–165 calories each

Imperial (Metric)
14 oz (400g) can cannellini beans
4 oz (100g) cracked wheat or
  burghul
1 vegetable stock cube
1 onion, diced
2 cloves garlic, crushed
1 tablespoonful vegetable oil
2 oz (50g) wholemeal breadcrumbs
1 carrot, grated
2 oz (50g) hazelnuts, toasted and
  chopped
1 teaspoonful dried mint

American
2 cupsful cooked beans
½ cupful burghul
1 vegetable stock cube
1 onion, diced
2 cloves garlic, crushed
1 tablespoonful vegetable oil
1 cupful wholewheat breadcrumbs
1 carrot, grated
½ cupful ground hazelnuts
1 teaspoonful dried mint

1. Lightly oil a baking tray and set the oven to 400°F/200°C (Gas Mark 6).

2. Drain the beans and place in a food processor.

3. Boil the cracked wheat in twice its volume of water with the stock cube for ten minutes then add to the processor.

4. While the grain is cooking sauté the onion and garlic in the oil until soft then add this to the processor.

5. Blend to a thick purée adding the breadcrumbs to make a firm paste.

6. Take small handfuls of the paste and mould a cavity into them to make a shell and place a dessertspoonful of the combined carrot, nut and mint in the centre then work around more paste to completely encase.

7. Bake for 25 minutes. Serve hot or cold.

BROWN RICE RING

Serves 4.
4½g fibre/400 calories per portion.

Imperial (Metric)	American
¾ lb (350g) brown rice	1½ cupsful brown rice
1 red pepper	1 red pepper
1 yellow pepper	1 yellow pepper
1 oz (25g) sunflower seeds	¼ cupful sunflower seeds
2 oz (50g) pine kernels	½ cupful pine kernels

1. Place the washed rice in a saucepan of boiling water and cook until soft — about 40 minutes.

2. Scrub and finely dice the peppers.

3. Put the rice in a mixing bowl when cooked and stir in the diced peppers. Add the sunflower seeds and pine kernels.

4. Rinse a savarin mould with cold water and pour water away.

5. Press the rice mixture into the wet mould. By pressing the mixture down firmly the rice will take shape when the mould is removed.

6. Chill in the fridge before use.

7. To unmould, place a serving dish on top of mould and invert, supporting plate. If the rice does not come away easily slip a palette knife around sides, invert and tap the top gently when inverted.

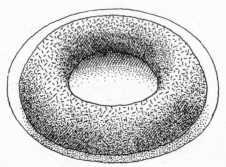

PARSNIP CHEESE
Serves 4.
7g fibre/350 calories per portion.

Imperial (Metric)	**American**
2 lb (1 kilo) parsnips	2 pounds parsnips
2 oz (50g) unsalted butter or polyunsaturated margarine	¼ cupful unsalted butter or polyunsaturated margarine
4 oz (100g) wholemeal breadcrumbs	2 cupsful wholewheat breadcrumbs
4 oz (100g) mature English Cheddar cheese	1 cupful hard cheese of choice

1. Scrub the parsnips and chop roughly.

2. Put them in a large saucepan and boil or steam until just cooked.

3. Drain and mash with a potato masher, mixing in margarine or butter.

4. Stir in the breadcrumbs and cheese and place in a lightly oiled ovenproof dish.

5. Make a pattern on top with a fork and grill for a few minutes, or bake in a moderate oven, until top is golden brown and mixture has heated through.

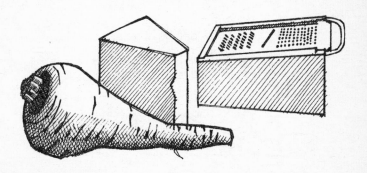

PARSNIP AND TOMATO BAKE *Illustrated in colour*

Serves 4.

7g fibre/500 calories per portion.

Imperial (Metric)	American
2 lb (1 kilo) parsnips	2 pounds parsnips
1 lb (½ kilo) tomatoes	1 pound tomatoes
2 oz (50g) unsalted butter or polyunsaturated margarine	¼ cupful unsalted butter or polyunsaturated margarine
Sea salt	Sea salt
Freshly ground black pepper	Freshly ground black pepper
6 oz (100g) Edam or 4 oz (100g) Gruyère cheese, grated	1½ cupsful Edam or 1 cupful Gruyère cheese, grated
¼ pint (150ml) single cream	⅔ cupful light cream
2 oz (50g) wholemeal breadcrumbs	1 cupful wholewheat breadcrumbs

1. Scrub the parsnips and cut into strips.

2. Place in a lightly oiled pan with well fitting lid and sweat for 5 minutes.

3. Place the tomatoes in boiling water for 1 minute. Drain and transfer to cold water. Slit the skins which should now be easily removed. Slice tomatoes thinly.

4. Lightly oil an ovenproof dish with some of the fat.

5. Put a layer of parsnips in the base, cover with a layer of tomatoes. Season and sprinkle with a little cheese and cream.

6. Repeat layers, reserving a little cheese. Mix the cheese with breadcrumbs and use as topping.

7. Bake at 350°F/180°C (Gas Mark 4) for 40 minutes.

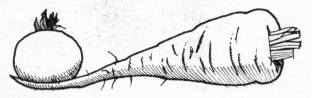

CHICKPEA AND MARROW HOTPOT
Serves 4.
9½g fibre/500 calories per portion.

Imperial (Metric)
½ lb (¼ kilo) hummous (page 44, halve the quantities)
1 marrow
1 lb (½ kilo) new potatoes
1 bunch spring onions
4 carrots

American
1 cupful hummous (page 44, halve the quantities)
1 summer squash
1 pound new potatoes
1 bunch scallions
4 carrots

1. Wash the marrow (summer squash) and slice into thick rounds.

2. Lightly oil a large casserole and arrange the marrow rings inside.

3. Fill the rings with hummus.

4. Scrub the potatoes and place, whole, around the marrow rings.

5. Wash and trim the onions and add to the casserole.

6. Scrub the carrots and place in the casserole with two or three tablespoonsful water.

7. Cover and bake at 375°F/190°C (Gas Mark 5) for 30 minutes.

Note: It should not be necessary to add more water or vegetable stock because the marrow (summer squash) will produce its own and will cook in its own steam. However, check during cooking to make sure the dish is not burning and add water or stock if necessary.

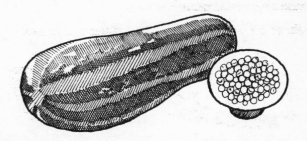

LEEK PIE
Serves 4
5.5 grams fibre/250 calories per serving

Imperial (Metric)	American
1 lb (450g) leeks	1 pound leeks
2 free range eggs	2 free range eggs
2 oz (50g) mature Cheddar cheese	1 cupful grated Cheddar cheese
¼ pint (150ml) natural yogurt	⅔ cupful natural yogurt
Freshly ground black pepper	Freshly ground black pepper
Sea salt	Sea salt

Pastry:

Imperial (Metric)	American
3 oz (75g) wholemeal flour	¾ cupful wholewheat flour
Sea salt	Sea salt
1 oz (25g) porridge oats	¼ cupful porridge oats
2 oz (50g) soft vegetable margarine	¼ cupful soft vegetable margarine

1. Lightly oil a pie dish and set the oven to 400°F/200°C (Gas Mark 6).

2. Trim the leeks and cut into 1 inch (2.5cm) slices then wash thoroughly. Boil for five minutes and drain, place in the base of the pie dish.

3. Beat the eggs with the cheese, yogurt and seasoning and pour over the leeks.

4. Make the pastry by sieving the flour and salt into the bowl, stirring in the oats and then rubbing in the fat until the mixture resembles breadcrumbs in consistency.

5. Add enough water to make a soft dough and roll out to cover the top of the pie dish, leaving an extra 1 inch (2.5cm) all round which is to be cut off and placed on the pie dish to make a pie rim.

6. Glaze with milk or beaten egg and fix the lid on top, then glaze the top and pierce a hole in the lid before baking for 30 minutes or until golden brown and crispy.

TOMATO BEAN BALLS

Serves 4.
6g fibre/250 calories per portion.

Imperial (Metric)	American
4 oz (100g) cooked blackeye beans	1 cupful cooked blackeye beans
4 oz (100g) ground hazelnuts	1 cupful ground hazelnuts
1 tablespoonful tahini	1 tablespoonful tahini
1 thick slice wholemeal bread	1 thick slice wholewheat bread
½ lb (¼ kilo) tinned tomatoes	1 small can tomatoes
Sea salt	Sea salt
Freshly ground black pepper	Freshly ground black pepper
1 orange	1 orange
1 tablespoonful tomato *purée*	1 tablespoonful tomato paste

1. Place the beans in a food processor with the nuts and tahini.

2. Make breadcrumbs from the slice of bread and add to beans.

3. Drain tinned tomatoes and add the fruit only to the food processor, reserve the juice. Blend all the ingredients in the food processor.

4. Remove from processor and season to taste. Add grated rind of well-washed orange.

5. Form the bean mixture into balls and place on a lightly oiled baking tray. Bake at 400°F/200°C (Gas Mark 6) for 30 minutes.

6. To make the sauce place juice from tinned tomatoes, juice from orange and tomato *purée* in saucepan. Heat through and dilute, if preferred, with water.

7. Pour the sauce over the hot bean balls and serve at once.

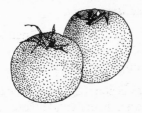

PASTA NIÇOISE
Serves 2.
4½g fibre/145 calories per portion.

Imperial (Metric)	American
½ red pepper	½ red pepper
1 clove garlic	1 clove garlic
3 shallots	3 shallots
4 tomatoes	4 tomatoes
4 oz (100g) wholemeal pasta shells	2 cupsful wholewheat pasta shells
½ pint (¼ litre) water or vegetable stock	1¼ cupsful water or vegetable stock
1 oz (25g) black olives	¼ cupful black olives
1 tablespoonful freshly chopped parsley	1 tablespoonful freshly chopped parsley
1 tablespoonful freshly chopped chives	1 tablespoonful freshly chopped chives
1 tablespoonful tomato ketchup	1 tablespoonful tomato catsup
1 small can anchovy fillets	1 small can anchovy fillets

1. Wash and dice the red pepper. Place in a lightly oiled saucepan.

2. Crush the garlic, dice shallots and chop the tomatoes and add to saucepan. Cover and cook over low heat for 5 minutes.

3. While the vegetables are cooking, place the pasta in a saucepan of boiling water and cook for about 12 minutes or until *al dente* (still firm to the teeth when bitten, but just cooked).

4. Add stock to the tomato mixture and stir in the olives, herbs, ketchup and anchovies. Continue to cook for 5 minutes.

5. Drain the pasta and place in a serving dish. Pour on the tomato sauce and serve at once.

DOLMAS

Serves 4.
9g fibre/350 calories per portion.

Imperial (Metric)	American
8 large outer cabbage leaves	8 large outer leaves of cabbage
1 tablespoonful olive oil	1 tablespoonful olive oil
½ lb (¼ kilo) onion, diced	1⅓ cupful onion, diced
1 clove garlic, crushed	1 clove garlic, crushed
1 lb (450g) celeriac, diced	1 pound celeriac, diced
½ oz (12g) sunflower seeds	3½ tablespoonsful sunflower seeds
2 oz (50g) pine kernels	½ cupful pine kernels
2 oz (50g) sultanas	⅓ cupful golden seedless raisins
½ lb (¼ kilo) cooked brown rice	1⅓ cupful cooked brown rice
4 oz (100g) tomato sauce (page 104)	1¼ cupful tomato sauce (page 104)

1. Clean the cabbage leaves and blanch in boiling water. Drain, reserving liquid.

2. Place the oil in a saucepan and add the onion and garlic. *Sauté* for 5 minutes.

3. Add the celeriac and sunflower seeds. Cover and cook for 5 minutes over low heat.

4. Stir in pine kernels, sultanas and rice. Heat through.

5. Spread the cabbage leaves open on a clean work surface and divide mixture between the leaves. Fold the leaves around mixture and transfer to a lightly oiled ovenproof dish.

6. Pour tomato sauce over the stuffed leaves and bake at 425°F/220°C (Gas Mark 7) for 30 minutes.

CONTINENTAL LENTIL COTTAGE PIE

Serves 4.
8g fibre/330 calories per portion.

Imperial (Metric)	American
½ lb (¼ kilo) brown or continental lentils	1 cupful brown or continental lentils
1 bay leaf	1 bay leaf
1 leek, sliced	1 leek, sliced
2 carrots, sliced	2 carrots, sliced
1 onion, diced	1 onion, diced
1 teaspoonful vegetable stock concentrate	1 teaspoonful vegetable stock concentrate
1 tablespoonful wholemeal flour	1 tablespoonful wholewheat flour
1 lb (½ kilo) potatoes	1 pound potatoes
1 oz (25g) unsalted butter	2½ tablespoonsful unsalted butter
2½ fl oz (75ml) skimmed milk	⅓ cupful skimmed milk
1 free-range egg	1 free-range egg

1. Place the washed lentils in a saucepan with bay leaf. Cover with water and bring to the boil. Lower heat and simmer for 20 minutes.

2. Prepare the leek, carrots and onion and *sauté* in a frying pan (skillet) with a smear of oil.

3. When the lentils are cooked remove bay leaf and drain, if necessary. Add the vegetables to the lentils and stock concentrate.

4. Stir in a few tablespoonsful boiling water. Sprinkle on the flour and stir well until mixture thickens.

5. Transfer mixture to an ovenproof dish.

6. Meanwhile scrub the potatoes and boil. When cooked, mash and cool.

7. Transfer the potatoes to a liquidizer with the butter, milk and egg. Liquidize to smooth *purée* and spoon over the lentils.

8. Cover and bake at 400°F/200°C (Gas Mark 6) for 40 minutes.

RED LENTIL COTTAGE PIE

Serves 4.
10g fibre/350 calories per portion.

Imperial (Metric)	American
½ lb (¼ kilo) red lentils	1 cupful lentils
½ lb (¼ kilo) onion, diced	1⅓ cupsful diced onion
½ lb (¼ kilo) carrots, grated	1⅓ cupsful grated carrots
1 large green pepper	1 large green pepper
14 oz (400g) tin tomatoes	1 medium can tomatoes
Sea salt	Sea salt
Freshly ground black pepper	Freshly ground black pepper
1 lb (½ kilo) potatoes, boiled and mashed	2 cupsful potatoes, boiled and mashed
1 oz (25g) unsalted butter or polyunsaturated margarine	2½ tablespoonsful unsalted butter or polyunsaturated margarine
2 tablespoonsful skimmed milk	2 tablespoonsful skimmed milk

1. Pick over the lentils to remove any stones or grit. Wash well.

2. Place washed lentils in saucepan and cover with water. Bring to boil, lower heat and simmer for 20 minutes.

3. Put the lentils, onion, carrots, pepper and tomatoes in a saucepan and cook together for about 20 minutes. Break up the tomatoes with the back of a spoon to release their juice.

4. Mash fat and milk with potatoes. For smoother potatoes liquidize after mashing.

5. Stir together lentils and vegetable mixture, season and place in an ovenproof dish. Top with mashed potatoes and grill (broil) to brown or reheat if necessary.

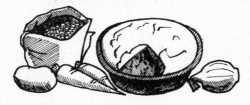

TOMATO SAUCE

Sauce contains 4g fibre and 55 calories.

Imperial (Metric)	American
1 lb (½ kilo) tomatoes, chopped	1 pound tomatoes, chopped
¼ pint (150ml) water	⅔ cupful water
Bunch parsley tied with string	Bunch parsley tied with string
1 bay leaf	1 bay leaf
Sprig thyme	Sprig thyme
2 sticks celery, roughly chopped	2 stalks celery, roughly chopped

1. Place all the ingredients in a heavy-based saucepan with well-fitting lid and simmer, covered, for 30 minutes.

2. Remove the bay leaf, thyme and parsley.

3. Place the rest of the ingredients in a liquidizer and blend to a smooth sauce.

9.

VEGETABLE SIDE DISHES

STUFFED TOMATOES *Illustrated in colour*
Serves 4.
5g fibre/150 calories each.

Imperial (Metric)	American
4 large beefsteak tomatoes	4 large beefsteak tomatoes
6 oz (150g) onion, diced	1 cupful diced onion
Clove garlic (optional)	Clove garlic (optional)
3 oz (75g) peanuts, finely chopped	½ cupful peanuts, finely chopped
1 stick celery, chopped	1 stalk celery, chopped
1 teaspoonful yeast extract	1 teaspoonful yeast extract
Few drops Tabasco	Few drops Tabasco
1 oz (25g) fresh wholemeal breadcrumbs	½ cupful fresh wholewheat breadcrumbs

1. Slice tops from the tomatoes and using serrated-edged teaspoon remove pips and pulp. Turn the tomatoes upside down to drain and place pips and pulp in saucepan.

2. Add the onion, garlic, peanuts and celery to tomato pulp and cook over a low heat for 5 minutes.

3. Stir in the yeast extract, Tabasco and breadcrumbs. Remove from heat and place the mixture in the tomatoes. Replace the tomato lids and hold in place with wooden cocktail sticks.

4. Place the stuffed tomatoes in a lightly oiled ovenproof dish and bake at 350°F/180°C (Gas Mark 4) for 20 minutes.

BAKED ONIONS

Serves 4.
5½g fibre/190 calories per portion.

Imperial (Metric)
4 large onions
4 oz (100g) cooked brown rice
4 oz (100g) roasted peanuts,
   chopped
1 medium-sized green pepper, diced
Sea salt
Freshly ground black pepper
¼ pint (150ml) vegetable stock

American
4 large onions
⅔ cupful cooked brown rice
¾ cupful roasted peanuts, chopped
1 medium-sized green pepper diced
Sea salt
Freshly ground black pepper
⅔ cupful vegetable stock

1. Steam or boil the onions in their skins for 20 minutes. Drain and allow to cool slightly.

2. Mix the cooked rice with nuts and pepper and season to taste.

3. Slice the top and bottom from onion and press out the centre of the onions, reserve. Place onions in an ovenproof dish.

4. Divide the rice mixture into 4 and fill the centre of the onions.

5. Finely chop the reserved onion and mix with stock. Pour over the onions.

6. Cover and bake at 400°F/200°C (Gas Mark 6) for 30 minutes.

BRAISED RED CABBAGE

Serves 4.
9g fibre/80 calories per portion.

Imperial (Metric)
2 lb (1 kilo) red cabbage
1 lb (½ kilo) cooking apples
1 tablespoonful Demerara sugar
¼ pint (150ml) red wine vinegar
¼ pint (150ml) water

American
2 pounds red cabbage
1 pound cooking apples
1 tablespoonful Demerara sugar
⅔ cupful red wine vinegar
⅔ cupful water

1. Shred the cabbage and wash well. Place in a large saucepan, or ovenproof dish (with well-fitting lid).

2. Wash and grate or slice the apples, but do not peel. Add to the cabbage.

3. Add the sugar and pour over the vinegar and water.

4. Cook on top of the stove over gentle heat for 30 minutes or bake at 350°F/180°C (Gas Mark 4) for 40 minutes.

RATATOUILLE

Serves 4.
4g fibre/98 calories per portion.

Imperial (Metric)	American
1 tablespoonful olive oil	1 tablespoonful olive oil
½ lb (¼ kilo) onion, peeled and diced	1⅓ cupsful peeled and diced onion
2 clove garlic, crushed	2 cloves garlic, crushed
½ lb (¼ kilo) aubergines, sliced	8 ounces eggplants, sliced
½ lb (¼ kilo) courgettes, sliced	8 ounces zucchini, sliced
½ lb (¼ kilo) green pepper, de-seeded and sliced	8 ounces green pepper, de-seeded and sliced
½ lb (¼ kilo) tomatoes, skinned and chopped	8 ounces tomatoes, skinned and chopped
2 tablespoonsful parsley, chopped	2 tablespoonsful parsley, chopped

1. Put the olive oil in a large heavy-based saucepan. Add the onion and garlic and *sauté* for 3 minutes.

2. Add the rest of the vegetables and stir together well. Cover and leave to simmer for about 40 minutes, stirring occasionally to prevent sticking.

3. Alternatively place mixture in an ovenproof dish with well-fitting lid and bake at 350°F/180°C (Gas Mark 4) for about 1 hour.

4. Before serving sprinkle with parsley and stir in.

SPINACH CHOUX BALLS
Makes 10.
4½g fibre/300 calories per ball.

Imperial (Metric)
10 oz (300g) wholemeal flour
¾ pint (400ml) water
4 oz (100g) unsalted butter or
    polyunsaturated margarine
3 free-range egg yolks
½ teaspoonful cayenne pepper

American
2½ cupsful wholewheat flour
2 cupsful water
½ cupful unsalted butter or
    polyunsaturated margarine
3 free-range egg yolks
½ teaspoonful cayenne pepper

Filling:

Imperial (Metric)
4 oz (100g) unsalted butter or
    polyunsaturated margarine
4 oz (100g) wholemeal flour
1 pint (½ litre) vegetable stock
½ lb (¼ kilo) frozen spinach or
    1 lb (½ kilo) fresh spinach
4 oz (100g) quark, or similar low-fat,
    soft white cheese

American
½ cupful unsalted butter or
    polyunsaturated margarine
1 cupful wholewheat flour
2½ cupsful vegetable stock
1 cupful frozen spinach or
    2 cupsful fresh spinach
½ cupful quark, or similar low-fat,
    soft white cheese

1. Place the water and fat in a saucepan and bring to boiling point.

2. Remove from heat and beat in the sieved flour.

3. Gradually beat in the egg yolks one at a time until the mixture is smooth and shiny and leaves the sides of the pan in one lump.

4. Place pastry in a piping bag with ¾ in. (2cm) plain nozzle and pipe 20 balls onto a lightly oiled baking tray.

5. Bake at 425°F/220°C (Gas Mark 7) for about 20 minutes, or until balls are golden brown and well risen and inserted skewer comes out clean.

6. To make the filling place butter and flour in saucepan over low heat and stir to make a *roux* (thick paste).

7. Gradually add stock, stirring continuously to form a thick, smooth sauce.

8. Remove from heat and stir in finely chopped spinach. Cool.

9. Stir in the cheese and place in a piping bag with ¼ in. (5mm) plain nozzle.

10. Insert nozzle into base of choux balls and fill with spinach mixture.

TURNIP PURÉE
Serves 4.
11g fibre/150 calories per portion.

Imperial (Metric)	American
2 lb (1 kilo) small turnips	2 pounds small turnips
1 lb (½ kilo) carrots	1 pound carrots
Pinch sea salt	Pinch sea salt
1 oz (25g) unsalted butter, or polyunsaturated margarine	2½ tablespoonsful unsalted butter, or polyunsaturated margarine
Freshly ground black pepper	Freshly ground black pepper
2 tablespoonsful soured cream	2 tablespoonsful soured cream
Freshly chopped chervil to garnish	Freshly chopped chervil to garnish

1. Scrub and dice the turnips, do not peel.

2. Scrub and dice the carrots, do not peel.

3. Place the turnips and carrots in a vegetable steamer or boil in the minimum of water until just cooked. Drain, reserving cooking liquid.

4. Add seasoning, butter, and soured cream and mash with a potato masher. For a finer *purée* place the mashed vegetables in a liquidizier or food processor and blend.

5. Return to saucepan with a little of the reserved cooking liquid and reheat quickly before serving.

6. Garnish with chervil.

CARROT SWEDE PURÉE

Serves 4.
12g fibre/160 calories per portion.

Imperial (Metric)
2 lb (1 kilo) swede, scrubbed and
    diced
1 lb (½ kilo) carrots, scrubbed and
    sliced
Sea salt
Freshly ground black pepper
1 oz (25g) unsalted butter, or
    polyunsaturated margarine
2 tablespoonsful soured cream
Freshly chopped parsley to garnish

American
2 pounds rutabaga, scrubbed and
    diced
1 pound carrots, scrubbed and sliced
Sea salt
Freshly ground black pepper
2½ tablespoonsful unsalted butter or
    polyunsaturated margarine
2 tablespoonsful soured cream
Freshly chopped parsley to garnish

1. Scrub and dice the swede (rutabaga), do not peel.

2. Scrub and dice the carrots, do not peel.

3. Place the swede (rutabaga) and carrots in a vegetable steamer or boil in minimum of water until just cooked. Drain, reserving cooking liquid.

4. Add seasoning, butter and soured cream and mash with potato masher. For finer *purée* place mashed vegetables in liquidizer or food processor and blend.

5. Return to saucepan with a little of the reserved cooking liquid and reheat quickly before serving.

6. Garnish with parsley.

10.

DESSERTS

BROWN BREAD ICE CREAM
Makes 6 scoops
1.5 grams fibre/115 calories per scoop

Imperial (Metric)
4 oz (100g) wholemeal breadcrumbs
2 oz (50g) Demerara sugar
½ pint (300ml) strained natural
   yogurt
3 drops natural vanilla essence
2 free range egg whites

American
2 cupsful wholewheat breadcrumbs
⅓ cupful Demerara sugar
1¼ cupsful thick natural yogurt
3 drops natural vanilla essence
2 free range egg whites

1. Mix together the breadcrumbs and the sugar and place in a grill pan and toast well, stirring from time to time, until browned and giving off a delicious aroma. Remove and cool.

2. Place the yogurt in a basin and stir in the vanilla and the cooled breadcrumbs mixture.

3. Whisk the egg whites until stiff and then fold into the mixture. Transfer to a shallow tray and freeze, breaking up with a fork when on the point of freezing and then transferring to a container which is deep enough to allow you to take scoops of the mixture when ready to serve. Or prepare in an ice cream maker.

4. Before serving ice cream remove from the freezer and allow it to soften slightly in a fridge for 20–30 minutes.

JACK HORNER CRUMBLE

Serves 4.
14g fibre/400 calories per portion.

Imperial (Metric)	American
½ lb (¼ kilo) prunes	2 cupsful prunes
½ lb (¼ kilo) fresh plums	2 cupsful fresh plums
2 large cooking apples	2 large cooking apples
6 oz (150g) wholemeal flour	1½ cupsful wholewheat flour
½ teaspoonful mixed spice	½ teaspoonful mixed spice
3 oz (75g) polyunsaturated margarine	⅓ cupful polyunsaturated margarine
2 oz (50g) Demerara sugar	⅓ cupful Demerara sugar

1. Soak the prunes overnight in boiling water. Cook in boiling water for about 30 minutes, or until soft enough to remove stones.

2. Halve the plums and remove stones.

3. Core and thinly slice the unpeeled apple. Place in the saucepan with plums and heat gently for about 5 minutes, until juices run from the plums.

4. Lightly oil an ovenproof dish. Mix fruit together and place in dish. Add a couple of tablespoonsful of water.

5. Sieve the flour and spice into a separate bowl and add the fat.

6. Rub fat into flour until the mixture resembles breadcrumbs in texture.

7. Stir in the sugar and place on top of the fruit. Bake at 400°F/200°C (Gas Mark 6) for about 40 minutes.

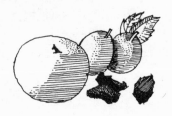

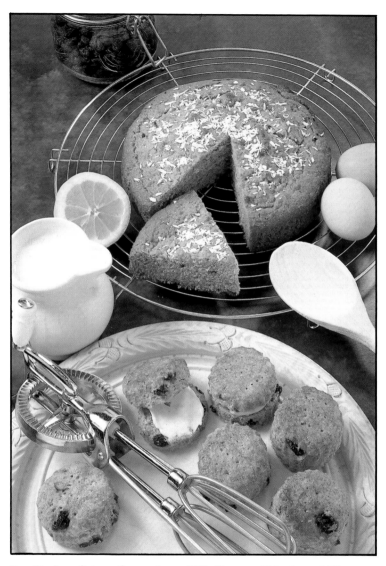

7. Teatime: Sultana Scones (page 132); Coconut Cake (page 139).

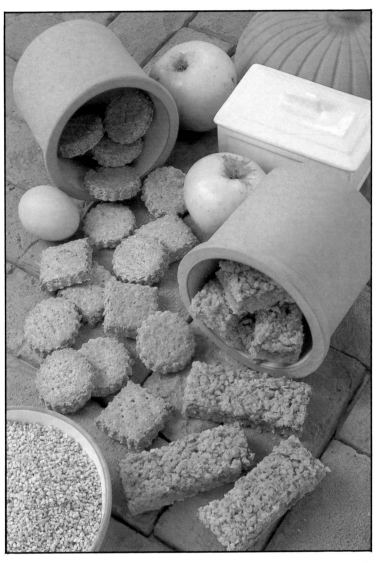

8.   Oaty Treats: Oatmeal Biscuits (page 135) and Date Flapjacks (page 141).

AUTUMN PUDDING

Serves 4.
18g fibre/300 calories per portion.

Imperial (Metric)
½ lb (¼ kilo) elderberries
½ lb (¼ kilo) blackberries
1 lb (½ kilo) cooking apples
¼ pint (150ml) water
1 small wholemeal loaf

American
2 cupsful elderberries
2 cupsful blackberries
1 pound cooking apples
⅔ cupful water
1 small wholewheat loaf

1. Wash the elderberries and pull from stems. Place in a saucepan.

2. Wash and pick over the blackberries. Add to elderberries. Cover and cook over gentle heat for 10 minutes.

3. Core and slice the unpeeled apples and place in another saucepan with water. Cook until soft and beat to a pulp.

4. Line 1½ pint (¾ litre) pudding basin with slices of bread trimmed to fit.

5. Mix together the fruits, reserving any juice and pour into the basin.

6. Place more bread on top of the fruit and pour over the reserved juice to soak bread thoroughly.

7. Place a saucer that fits inside the top of the basin in position and place weights on it to press it down. Leave overnight in fridge. Unmould before serving.

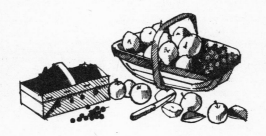

PRUNE JELLIES

Serves 4.
20g fibre/210 calories per portion.

Imperial (Metric)	American
1 lb (½ kilo) prunes	4 cupsful prunes
½ pint (¼ litre) red wine	1¼ cupsful red wine
¼ pint (150ml) water	⅔ cupful water
1 orange	1 orange
½ lb (¼ kilo) redcurrants	2 cupsful redcurrants
½ oz (15g) gelatine or agar-agar	2 teaspoonsful gelatine or agar-agar

1. Place the prunes in a saucepan with the wine, water and rind of well-washed orange and bring to boil. Lower heat and simmer with lid on for 40 minutes or until prunes are cooked.

2. Top and tail the currants and place in another saucepan over a low heat. Cook for about 5 minutes. Remove and rub through sieve.

3. Soak the gelatine in the orange juice.

4. When the prunes are cooked strain the hot liquid onto gelatine, stirring all the time until the gelatine or agar-agar has dissolved.

5. Discard the orange rind and place prunes in bottom of individual glass dishes.

6. Add the redcurrant juice to the prune juice and leave to cool. When on point of setting pour over prunes.

7. Place jellies in the fridge to cool before serving.

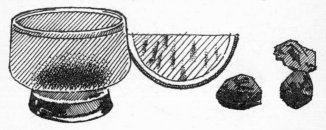

HOT FRUIT COMPOTE
Serves 4.
10g fibre/155 calories per portion.

Imperial (Metric)	American
1 pint (½ litre) water	2½ cupsful water
1 tablespoonful clear honey	1 tablespoonful clear honey
1 teaspoonful cinnamon	1 teaspoonful cinnamon
1 teaspoonful nutmeg	1 teaspoonful nutmeg
2 cloves	2 cloves
1 lemon	1 lemon
4 oz (100g) dried apricots	1 cupful dried apricots
14 oz (400g) tin peaches tinned in own, or apple juice	1 medium can peaches, canned in own juice or apple juice
4 oz (100g) sultanas	⅔ cupful golden seedless raisins

1. Place the water, honey, spices and juice and grated rind of well-washed lemon in a saucepan and bring to boil.

2. Add the apricots and reduce heat. Cover and simmer for 30 minutes.

3. Add the peaches and sultanas (golden seedless raisins) and cook for further 10 minutes.

4. Serve hot. Offer natural yogurt separately.

Note: Any left-over *compote* is nice for breakfast on its own or with natural unsweetened yogurt.

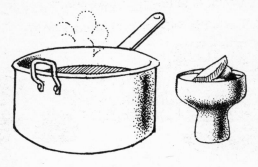

CHRISTMAS PUDDING

Serves 8.
6g fibre/450 calories per portion.

Imperial (Metric)	American
½ lb (¼ kilo) raisins	1⅓ cupsful raisins
1 lemon, rind and juice	1 lemon, rind and juice
1 orange, rind and juice	1 orange, rind and juice
2 oz (50g) blanched almonds, finely chopped	½ cupful blanched almonds, finely chopped
4 oz (100g) currants	⅔ cupful currants
4 oz (100g) sultanas	⅔ cupful golden seedless raisins
2 oz (50g) wholemeal flour	½ cupful wholewheat flour
Pinch each of ground nutmeg, mixed spice, ground cinnamon,	Pinch each of ground nutmeg, mixed spice and ground cinnamon,
4 oz (100g) wholemeal breadcrumbs	1 cupful wholewheat breadcrumbs
½ lb (¼ kilo) unsalted butter or polyunsaturated margarine	2 cupsful unsalted butter or polyunsaturated margarine
2 tablespoonsful brandy	2 tablespoonsful brandy
3 free-range eggs	3 free-range eggs

1. Mix together all the dry ingredients.

2. Warm together in a saucepan the lemon juice, orange juice, butter and brandy. Remove from heat.

3. Beat the eggs well and add to the other liquids. Stir into dry ingredients.

4. Mixture should have a soft dropping consistency (drops easily from a raised spoon). If dry add more liquid, such as milk, water or juice.

5. Fill lightly oiled pudding basin with mixture, leaving about 1½ ins. (4cm) at the top to allow for rising.

6. Cover basin with pleated double layer of oiled greaseproof paper topped with aluminium foil or a pudding cloth, tied beneath the rim with string.

7. Set basin in a large pan of boiling water or a steamer, or place in a pressure cooker.

8. Steam for 6 hours, topping up with boiling water as necessary. If using a pressure cooker steam according to manufacturer's instructions.

9. Allow to cool and store. Before serving on Christmas Day steam for a further 2 hours.

SUMMER PUDDING
Serves 4.
13g fibre/290 calories per portion.

Imperial (Metric)	American
½ lb (¼ kilo) raspberries	2½ cupsful raspberries
½ lb (¼ kilo) redcurrants	2½ cupsful redcurrants
½ lb (¼ kilo) blackcurrants	2½ cupsful blackcurrants
Small wholemeal loaf	Small wholewheat loaf

1. Wash the fruit and top and tail currants.

2. Place fruit in a saucepan over a low heat. Cover and cook for 2 or 3 minutes only, until juices begin to run from the fruit.

3. Remove pan from heat and set aside.

4. Thinly slice the loaf, and line a pudding basin with the bread. Trim bread to fit.

5. Pour fruit and juice into the lined pudding basin and cover the fruit with more slices of bread.

6. Find a saucer that fits just inside the rim of the basin and place it on top of the bread and fruit.

7. Place a weight on top of the saucer and chill for several hours before inverting to remove from basin and serving.

PEACH GALETTE

Serves 4.
11g fibre/550 calories per portion.

Imperial (Metric)	American
½ lb (¼ kilo) dried peaches	2 cupsful dried peaches
4 oz (100g) unsalted butter, or polyunsaturated margarine	½ cupful unsalted butter, or polyunsaturated margarine
3 oz (75g) oatbran and oatgerm	¾ cupful oatbran and oatgerm
3 oz (75g) rolled oats	¾ cupful rolled oats
1 free-range egg	1 free-range egg
¼ pint (150ml) quark, or *fromage blanc*	½ cupful quark, or *fromage blanc*

1. Place the dried peaches in a saucepan and cover with boiling water. Place lid on saucepan and simmer for about 30 minutes until soft. Drain and *purée* in liquidizer.

2. Beat together half the *purée* (reserving half for filling) with the butter or margarine.

3. Add the oatbran and oatgerm and rolled oats.

4. Beat in the egg.

5. Place the mixture in a piping bag with ¾ in. (2cm) plain nozzle and pipe 3 rounds, each 6 in. (15cm) in diameter, on lightly oiled baking tray.

6. Bake at 375°F/190°C (Gas Mark 5) for 25-30 minutes until firm to touch and golden brown. Remove from oven and cool.

7. Mix together remaining *purée* and quark or *fromage blanc*.

8. Sandwich the 3 galette layers together with the dried peach and cheese *purée*.

RHUBARB FOOL
Serves 4.
7g fibre/215 calories per portion.

Imperial (Metric)
1 lb (½ kilo) rhubarb, sliced into
   1 in. (2cm) pieces
1 tablespoonful honey
1 teaspoonful ground cinnamon
1 lb (½ kilo) bananas
½ pint (¼ litre) thick-set natural
   yogurt
2 oz (50g) wheatgerm
2 oz (50g) hazelnuts, chopped

American
1 pound rhubarb, sliced into
   1 in. pieces
1 tablespoonful honey
1 teaspoonful ground cinnamon
1 pound bananas
1¼ cupsful thick-set natural yogurt
½ cupful wheatgerm
½ cupful hazelnuts, chopped

1. Wash and slice the rhubarb. Place in a saucepan with honey, cinnamon and 6 tablespoonsful of water. Cover and cook over low heat for about 15 minutes.

2. Place the peeled and chopped bananas in a liquidizer and blend to *purée*.

3. Add yogurt and mix thoroughly.

4. Add cooled rhubarb and mix again.

5. Turn into individual serving dishes.

6. Before serving top with wheatgerm and nuts.

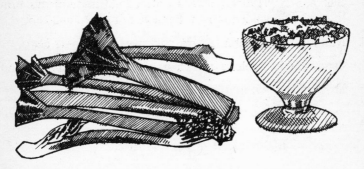

BAKEWELL TART *Illustrated in colour*
Serves 6
4.5 grams fibre/400 calories per portion

Pastry:

Imperial (Metric)	American
6 oz (150g) wholemeal flour	1½ cupsful wholewheat flour
2½ oz (70g) soft vegetable margarine	⅓ cupful margarine
Water to mix	Water to mix

Filling:

Imperial (Metric)	American
4 oz (100g) soft vegetable margarine	½ cupful margarine
4 oz (100g) muscovado sugar	⅔ cupful sugar
2 free range eggs	2 free range eggs
2 drops natural almond essence	2 drops natural almond essence
4 oz (100g) wholemeal flour	1 cupful wholewheat flour
2 tablespoonsful no added sugar jam	2 tablespoonsful no added sugar jam

1. Sift the flour into a mixing bowl and rub in the fat until the mixture resembles breadcrumbs in consistency, then mix in enough cold water to make a soft dough.

2. Roll out on a lightly floured board and line a 7 in. (17.5cm) baking dish or flan tin.

3. Cream the margarine and sugar together and beat in the eggs, one at a time until the mixture is light and creamy. Add the essence.

4. Sift the flour and fold into the mixture.

5. Spread the jam on the bottom of the pastry case and then spoon the sponge mixture on top. Smooth the top and make a lattice with any left over pieces of pastry, if liked.

6. Bake in a pre-set oven at 400°F/200°C (Gas Mark 6) for 40 minutes or until the sponge is set and the bakewell tart is golden brown in colour.

APRICOT AND COCONUT CRUMBLE

Serves 6.
18g fibre/300 calories per portion.

Imperial (Metric)
4 oz (100g) dried apricots
4 oz (100g) raisins
2 oz (50g) sultanas
4 oz (100g) peaches, tinned in own
  or apple juice

American
1 cupful dried apricots
2/3 cupful raisins
1/3 cupful golden seedless raisins
1 cupful peaches, canned in own or
  apple juice

Topping:

Imperial (Metric)
3 oz (75g) wholemeal flour
3 oz (75g) rolled oats
3 oz (75g) polyunsaturated
  margarine
2 oz (50g) ground coconut
2 oz (50g) dates, chopped

American
3/4 cupful wholewheat flour
3/4 cupful rolled oats
1/3 cupful polyunsaturated margarine
2/3 cupful ground coconut
1/3 cupful dates, chopped

1. Place the apricots in a saucepan with boiling water and simmer for 40 minutes until soft. Cool and *purée*.

2. Stir in the sultanas (golden seedless raisins) and drained peaches. Place in an ovenproof dish and add a few tablespoonsful water.

3. Mix together the flour and oats.

4. Rub the margarine into the flour and oats and stir in the coconut and dates. Place on top of fruit.

5. Bake at 375°F/190°C (Gas Mark 5) for 30 minutes.

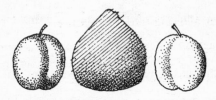

GOOSEBERRY CHEESECAKE

Serves 6.
4½g fibre/320 calories per portion.

Pastry:

Imperial (Metric)	American
6 oz (150g) wholemeal flour	1½ cupsful wholewheat flour
4 oz (100g) polyunsaturated margarine	½ cupful polyunsaturated margarine
Water to mix	Water to mix

Filling:

Imperial (Metric)	American
4 oz (100g) gooseberries	1 cupful gooseberries
2 tablespoonsful clear honey	2 tablespoonsful clear honey
5 oz (125g) cottage cheese	⅔ cupful cottage cheese
1 free-range egg, separated	1 free-range egg, separated
1 oz (25g) ground almonds	¼ cupful ground almonds
1 oz (25g) wholemeal semolina	¼ cupful wholewheat semolina
1 free-range egg white	1 free-range egg white
2 oz (50g) raisins, soaked in liqueur	⅓ cupful raisins, soaked in liqueur

1. Sieve the flour into a mixing bowl.

2. Rub fat into flour until the mixture resembles breadcrumbs in texture.

3. Form a soft dough by adding water.

4. Roll out on a lightly floured surface and carefully lift into base of a lightly oiled 8 in. (20cm) cake tin or flan ring.

5. Top and tail the gooseberries and place in a saucepan with 2 tablespoonsful water. Cover and simmer for about 15 minutes. Cool and *purée*.

6. Beat together the honey, cheese, egg yolk, almonds and semolina.

7. Add the cooled gooseberries.

8. Whisk the egg whites to firm peaks and quickly fold into mixture.

9. Place the raisins on the base of prepared pastry and pour over the gooseberry mixture.

10. Bake at 350°F/180°C (Gas Mark 4) for 40 minutes, or until set and firm to touch.

DE LUXE FRUIT SALAD
Serves 4.
4g fibre/105 calories per portion.

Imperial (Metric)	American
1 nectarine	1 nectarine
1 dessert pear	1 dessert pear
1 peach	1 peach
1 Worcester apple, or other crisp English eating apple	1 Worcester apple, or crisp eating apple with white flesh and red skin
1 banana	1 banana
2 oranges	2 oranges
¼ pint (150ml) orange juice	⅔ cupful orange juice
4 oz (100g) green grapes	4 ounces green grapes

1. Wash all the fruit well.

2. Place orange juice in a serving dish and slice or dice all fruit straight into the juice to prevent browning. Do not peel fruit (except oranges and banana), but core if necessary, and remove pips from grapes, if desired.

3. Reserve ¼ of each fruit for decoration.

4. Mix salad well.

5. To decorate, thinly slice each ¼ of fruit and arrange on top of the salad.

PASSION FRUIT SORBET

Serves 4.
4g fibre/140 calories per portion.

Imperial (Metric)	American
2 oz (50g) fructose (fruit sugar)	1/3 cupful fructose (fruit sugar)
1/4 pint (150ml) apple juice	2/3 cupful apple juice
9-10 passion fruits	9-10 passion fruits
Juice of 1/2 lemon	Juice of 1/2 lemon
2 free-range egg whites	2 free-range egg whites

1. Place the fructose and apple juice in saucepan over low heat and dissolve fructose. Remove and cool.

2. Cut the fruits in half and scoop out pippy pulp. Place in a bowl.

3. Add the lemon juice and fructose to pulp and pour mixture into a shallow tray or ice-cream maker and place in the freezer.

4. When the mixture is on point of setting remove and fold in stiffly beaten egg whites.

5. Place in a wetted and chilled container and return to freezer.

6. To serve use an ice-cream scoop to take sorbet from the container.

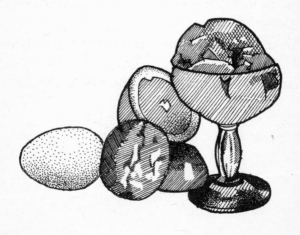

BLACKBERRY AND APPLE CRUMBLE

Serves 4.
8½g fibre/340 calories per portion.

Imperial (Metric)	American
1 lb (½ kilo) cooking apples	1 pound cooking apples
1 lemon	1 lemon
½ lb (¼ kilo) blackberries	8 ounces blackberries
2 oz (50g) wholemeal flour	½ cupful wholewheat flour
2 oz (50g) rolled oats	½ cupful rolled oats
3 oz (75g) unsalted butter or	½ cupful unsalted butter or
polyunsaturated margarine	polyunsaturated margarine
2 oz (50g) finely chopped dates	⅓ cupful finely chopped dates
1 oz (25g) sunflower seeds	¼ cupful sunflower seeds

1. Core and slice the unpeeled apples and dress with lemon juice to prevent browning. Place in saucepan with the washed blackberries.

2. Place over low heat and cover. Cook for 5 minutes.

3. Turn the fruit into a lightly oiled ovenproof dish.

4. Mix together the flour and oats.

5. Rub fat into the flour mixture until it resembles breadcrumbs in texture.

6. Stir in dates and sunflower seeds and place the mixture on top of the fruit.

7. Bake at 375°F/190°C (Gas Mark 5) for 30 minutes.

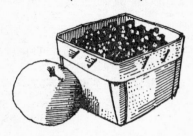

APRICOT GATEAU *Illustrated in colour*
Serves 6.
9g fibre/220 calories per portion.

Imperial (Metric)	American
3 free-range eggs	3 free-range eggs
3 oz (75g) clear honey	¼ cupful clear honey
1 tablespoonful boiling water	1 tablespoonful boiling water
3 oz (75g) wholemeal flour	⅔ cupful wholewheat flour

Topping:

Imperial (Metric)	American
8 oz (225g) dried apricots	1⅔ cupsful dried apricots
4 oz (100g) quark or similar low-fat, soft white cheese	½ cupful quark or similar low-fat, soft white cheese
4 oz (100g) thick-set natural yogurt	⅔ cupful thick-set natural yogurt

1. Whisk the eggs and honey until pale in colour and thick and ropey in texture.

2. Add water and quickly fold in the sieved wholemeal flour (and any bran left in the sieve) using a metal spoon.

3. Pour the mixture into a lightly oiled and lined 8 in. (20cm) cake tin.

4. Bake at 425°F/220°C (Gas Mark 7) for 15 minutes until golden brown and firm to the touch.

5. Remove from oven and leave in tin on wire baking tray to cool.

6. Cook the dried apricots in water until soft. Cool and *purée*.

7. Mix cold *purée* with cheese and yogurt.

8. Remove the cake from the tin, peel off paper. Using a palette knife carefully slice cake into 3 layers. Sandwich together with apricot *purée* and cover top and sides of gateau with rest of mixture.

11.

CAKES AND BAKES

HONEY AND HAZELNUT CAKE
Serves 4.
5g fibre/300 calories per portion.

Imperial (Metric)
4 free-range eggs, separated
½ lb (¼ kilo) clear honey
6 oz (150g) wholemeal flour
4 oz (100g) ground hazelnuts
3 fl oz (90ml) skimmed milk

American
4 free range eggs, separated
⅔ cupful clear honey
1½ cupsful wholewheat flour
1 cupful ground hazelnuts
⅓ cupful skimmed milk

1. Whisk egg yolks and honey until light and thick in texture.

2. Fold in sieved flour and hazelnuts.

3. Stir in milk.

4. Whisk egg whites until they form stiff peaks.

5. Fold egg whites into mixture and pour into lightly oiled and lined 8 in. (20cm) cake tin.

6. Bake at 350°F/180°C (Gas Mark 4) for 35-40 minutes or until golden brown and firm to touch.

CHRISTMAS CAKE

Serves 20, generously.
6g fibre/310 calories per portion.

Imperial (Metric)	American
½ lb (¼ kilo) wholemeal flour	2 cupsful wholewheat flour
1 teaspoonful mixed spice	1 teaspoonful mixed spice
1 teaspoonful ground nutmeg	1 teaspoonful ground nutmeg
1 teaspoonful ground cinnamon	1 teaspoonful ground cinnamon
1 teaspoonful ground cloves	1 teaspoonful ground cloves
4 oz (100g) ground almonds	1 cupful ground almonds
¾ lb (350g) currants	2 cupsful currants
¾ lb (350g) sultanas	2 cupsful golden seedless raisins
¾ lb (350g) raisins	2 cupsful raisins
6 oz (150g) blanched almonds, finely chopped	1½ cupsful blanched almonds, finely chopped
½ lb (¼ kilo) unsalted butter	2 cupsful unsalted butter
6 free-range eggs	6 free-range eggs
1 orange	1 orange
1 lemon	1 lemon
4 tablespoonsful brandy (optional)	⅓ cupful brandy (optional)

1. Sieve flour into mixing bowl with spices.

2. Stir in rest of dry ingredients.

3. In separate bowl cream butter and gradually add eggs. If mixture starts to separate add a little of the flour.

4. Stir butter and eggs into dry ingredients.

5. Scrub orange and lemon and grate rinds. Add the rinds and squeezed juice to the mixture.

6. If brandy is used stir it in.

7. Spoon mixture into 10 in. (25cm) oiled and lined cake tin and bake for 1½ hours at 300°F/150°C (Gas Mark 2), reduce heat to 250°F/130°C (Gas Mark ½) for a further 3 hours. Cover cake with brown or greaseproof paper or aluminium foil during the last 2 hours to prevent over-browning.

ROCK BUNS

Makes 12.
2g fibre/130 calories per bun

Imperial (Metric)
½ lb (¼ kilo) wholemeal flour
2 teaspoonsful baking powder
1 teaspoonful mixed spice or
   cinnamon
3 oz (75g) unsalted butter or
   polyunsaturated margarine
2 oz (50g) sultanas
2 oz (50g) currants
Grated rind of 1 lemon
3 fl oz (90ml) milk
1 free-range egg

American
2 cupsful wholewheat flour
2 teaspoonsful baking soda
1 teaspoonful mixed spice or
   cinnamon
⅓ cupful unsalted butter or
   polyunsaturated margarine
⅓ cupful golden seedless raisins
⅓ cupful currants
Grated rind of 1 lemon
⅓ cupful milk
1 free-range egg

1. Sieve the flour, baking powder and spice into mixing bowl.

2. Rub fat into flour until the mixture resembles breadcrumbs in texture.

3. Stir in the sultanas (golden seedless raisins), currants and lemon rind.

4. Stir milk into beaten egg and add to the dry ingredients to make them moist, but not sloppy.

5. Place a teaspoonful of mixture into lightly oiled bun tins or individual cake papers and roughen surface with a fork.

6. Bake at 400°F/200°C (Gas Mark 6) for 15 to 20 minutes.

Note: They are best eaten on the same day.

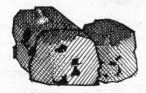

WHOLEMEAL BREAD

Loaf produces about 12 slices.
1½-2g fibre/50-55 calories per slice.

Imperial (Metric)
1 lb (½ kilo) wholemeal flour
Pinch sea salt
½ pint (¼ litre) water at 98°F
   (37°C) (blood heat)
½ oz (12g) fresh yeast, or
   1 oz (25g) dried
1 vitamin C tablet, crushed
1 tablespoonful corn oil
1 tablespoonful molasses

American
4 cupsful wholewheat flour
Pinch sea salt
1¼ cupsful water at 98°F (37°C)
   (blood heat)
1½ tablespoonsful fresh yeast, or
   1 tablespoonful dried
1 vitamin C tablet, crushed
1 tablespoonful corn oil
1 tablespoonful molasses

1. Sieve flour and salt together into bowl.

2. Place water in jug. The correct temperature can be achieved by using ⅓ boiling to ⅔ cold water.

3. Crumble yeast into water. Stir in crushed vitamin C tablet.

4. Add oil and molasses to yeast mixture and stir well.

5. Make a well in the centre of the flour and pour in liquid. Stir well to form a firm dough.

6. Turn onto lightly floured work surface and knead for 10 minutes. Knead by stretching dough away from the body using the heel of the hand. When stretched lift furthest point of dough back over body of dough and press again, away from body.

7. After kneading return dough to bowl and cover to prevent drying out and crust forming. Leave to rest for 10 minutes.

8. Heat oven to 425°F/220°C (Gas Mark 7) and lightly oil two small loaf tins.

9. Return risen dough to work surface and knead again. Form into sausage shape three times the width of the tin and fold two ends under. Place in tins and cover with a teatowel again to prevent crust forming. Leave in warm place until it has doubled in size.

10. Glaze with milk or beaten egg and bake for 45 minutes. Bread is ready when it falls easily from tins and sounds hollow when tapped on the base.

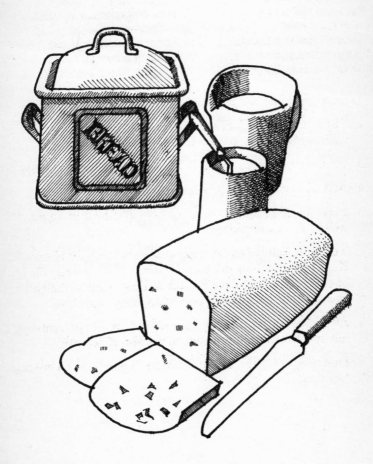

SULTANA SCONES *Illustrated in colour*
Makes one large round or 12 small scones.
23g fibre/1,160 calories, or
2g fibre/95 calories per scone.

Imperial (Metric)
½ lb (¼ kilo) wholemeal flour
1 teaspoonful baking powder
2 oz (50g) unsalted butter or
    polyunsaturated margarine
2 oz (50g) sultanas
¼ pint (150ml) buttermilk or
    skimmed milk with few drops of
    lemon juice added
Milk to glaze

American
2 cupsful wholewheat flour
1 teaspoonful baking powder
¼ cupful unsalted butter or
    polyunsaturated margarine
⅓ cupful golden seedless raisins
⅔ cupful buttermilk or skimmed milk
    with few drops of lemon juice
    added
Milk to glaze

1. Sieve the flour and baking powder into a bowl.

2. Rub the butter or margarine into the flour until the mixture resembles breadcrumbs in texture.

3. Stir the sultanas (golden seedless raisins) into mixture.

4. Make a well in the centre of the dry ingredients and gradually add milk, stirring to form a soft dough.

5. Turn the dough onto a lightly floured board and gently knead for a couple of minutes until dough holds its shape and is pliable.

6. Form into a large round and place on a baking tray. Alternatively roll out to ¾ in. (2cm) thickness and cut with pastry cutter into 12 scones.

7. Glaze with milk and bake at 450°F/230°C (Gas Mark 8) for 10 to 15 minutes.

SPICED TEABREAD PLAIT

Makes about 12 slices.
4g fibre/150 calories per slice.

Imperial (Metric)	American
6 oz (150g) sultanas	1 cupful golden seedless raisins
6 oz (150g) raisins	1 cupful raisins
½ pint (¼ litre) apple juice	1¼ cupsful apple juice
½ lb (¼ kilo) wholemeal flour	2 cupsful wholewheat flour
1 teaspoonful mixed spice	1 teaspoonful mixed spice
½ teaspoonful cinnamon	½ teaspoonful cinnamon
½ oz (12g) fresh yeast	1 tablespoonful fresh yeast
2 oz (50g) unsalted butter or polyunsaturated margarine	¼ cupful unsalted butter or polyunsaturated margarine
Apple juice, warmed	Apple juice, warmed

1. Soak the sultanas (golden seedless raisins) and raisins overnight in apple juice.

2. Sieve the flour and spices into a bowl and add bran from sieve.

3. Crumble yeast into flour.

4. Rub the margarine into the flour and yeast mixture.

5. Add the soaked fruit and warm juice to the flour mixture. Use only enough juice to make a firm dough.

6. Knead for 5 minutes on a floured surface. Return to bowl, cover and leave to rise.

7. When doubled in size knock back by kneading again for 2 minutes. Divide the dough into three pieces and roll into sausage shapes. Press one end of the three pieces together and plait the dough.

8. Lift dough onto lightly oiled baking tray and glaze with milk or beaten egg. Bake at 400°F/200°C (Gas Mark 6) for 30-40 minutes — until a skewer comes out cleanly.

BROWN BREAD PUDDING

Serves 12.
4g fibre/150 calories per portion.

Imperial (Metric)

½ large wholemeal loaf, broken up roughly

2 oz (50g) unsalted butter or polyunsaturated margarine

¼ pint (150ml) skimmed milk

2 oz (50g) clear honey

2 free-range eggs, beaten

4 oz (100g) sultanas and raisins

American

½ large wholewheat loaf, broken up roughly

¼ cupful unsalted butter or polyunsaturated margarine

⅔ cupful skimmed milk

2 tablespoonsful clear honey

2 free-range eggs, beaten

½ cupful golden seedless raisins and raisins

1. Soak the bread in cold water or milk for at least 30 minutes.

2. Squeeze moisture from bread.

3. Melt fat in a saucepan with milk and add to the broken-up bread.

4. Stir in the honey and beaten eggs and beat to a soggy pulp.

5. Stir in the fruit and place in a lightly oiled cake or baking tin.

6. Bake for 1 hour at 350°F/180°C (Gas Mark 4).

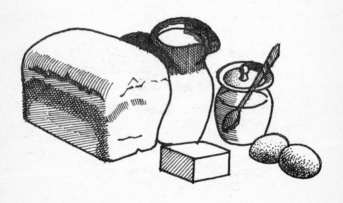

OATMEAL BISCUITS *Illustrated in colour*
Makes 30 biscuits.
1g fibre/52 calories per biscuit.

Imperial (Metric)	American
7 oz (200g) oatmeal	2 cupsful oatmeal
5 oz (125g) wholemeal flour	1¼ cupsful wholewheat flour
2 oz (50g) Demerara sugar	⅓ cupful Demerara sugar
1 teaspoonful baking powder	1 teaspoonful baking soda
4 oz (100g) unsalted butter, or	½ cupful unsalted butter, or
polyunsaturated margarine	polyunsaturated margarine
1 free-range egg	1 free-range egg
2 tablespoonsful skimmed milk	2 tablespoonsful skimmed milk

1. Mix together the oatmeal, flour, sugar and baking powder.

2. Rub in the fat to make a breadcrumb consistency.

3. Make a well in the centre of the ingredients and add the beaten egg and milk. Mix to a stiff dough.

4. Lightly flour a work surface and roll dough out thinly. Cut into biscuits with cutter.

5. Place biscuits on a lightly oiled baking tray and brush with milk or beaten egg. Bake at 375°F/190°C (Gas Mark 5) for 15 minutes until golden brown.

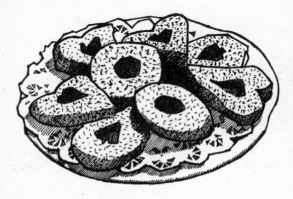

OATCAKES

Makes 20 oatcakes.
1g fibre/66 calories per oatcake.

Imperial (Metric)
½ lb (¼ kilo) oatmeal
2 oz (50g) wholemeal flour
1 teaspoonful baking powder
2 oz (50g) unsalted butter, or
   polyunsaturated margarine
Boiling water to mix

American
2 cupsful oatmeal
½ cupful wholewheat flour
1 teaspoonful baking soda
5 tablespoonsful butter, or
   polyunsaturated margarine
Boiling water to mix

1. Mix together the oatmeal, flour and baking powder.

2. Melt butter or margarine in a saucepan and stir into the dry ingredients.

3. Gradually add enough boiling water to make a dough, being careful not to add too much.

4. Knead lightly on a floured surface until the dough is firm enough to roll out.

5. Roll out and cut into triangles.

6. Slip a palette knife under oatcakes and carefully lift onto a lightly oiled baking tray. Sprinkle with a little oatmeal and bake at 375°F/190°C (Gas Mark 5) for about 10-15 minutes.

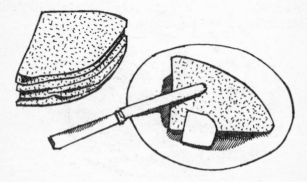

PRUNE DROPS

Makes about 20.
7g fibre/55 calories per drop.

Imperial (Metric)
4 oz (100g) prunes
2 oz (50g) unsalted butter or
   polyunsaturated margarine
1 tablespoonful clear honey
4 oz (100g) wholemeal flour
½ teaspoonful baking powder
1 free-range egg
1 oz (25g) flaked almonds

American
¾ cupful prunes
¼ cupful unsalted butter or
   polyunsaturated margarine
1 tablespoonful clear honey
1 cupful wholewheat flour
½ teaspoonful baking soda
1 free-range egg
¼ cupful slivered almonds

1. Wash the prunes and place in a saucepan. Cover with boiling water and cook until soft; about 40 minutes. Drain and cool before *puréeing* in liquidizer.

2. Cream together the prune *purée*, margarine and honey.

3. Add the sieved flour and baking powder, returning bran from sieve to mixture.

4. Beat in the free-range egg.

5. Place mixture in a piping bag with a star nozzle and pipe small drops onto a lightly oiled baking tray.

6. Place an almond on top of each drop and bake at 400°F/200°C (Gas Mark 6) for 15 minutes.

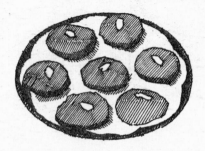

DATE AND PRUNE CAKE

Serves 8.
7g fibre/240 calories per portion.

Imperial (Metric)

4 oz (100g) unsalted butter or
  polyunsaturated margarine
2 oz (50g) clear honey
2 free-range eggs, beaten
6 oz (150g) wholemeal flour
2 teaspoonsful baking powder
1 teaspoonful cinnamon
1 teaspoonful mixed spice
½ lb (¼ kilo) prunes, stoned and
  soaked overnight in apple juice
4 oz (100g) dates, chopped
Water to mix

American

½ cupful unsalted butter or
  polyunsaturated margarine
¼ cupful clear honey
2 free-range eggs, beaten
1½ cupsful wholewheat flour
2 teaspoonsful baking soda
1 teaspoonful cinnamon
1 teaspoonful mixed spice
1½ cupsful prunes, stoned and
  soaked overnight in apple juice
¾ cupful chopped dates
Water to mix

1. Beat the margarine and honey together until light and fluffy.

2. Gradually add the eggs, beating continuously. If mixture shows signs of curdling add a little flour.

3. Sieve together the flour, baking powder and spices and fold into the margarine.

4. Chop the soaked prunes and add prunes and dates to mixture.

5. Add water, if required, to form a soft mixture.

6. Turn mixture into a lightly oiled 8 in. (20cm) cake tin and bake at 350°F/180°C (Gas Mark 4) for 1½ hours or until an inserted skewer comes out clean.

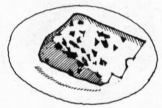

COCONUT CAKE *Illustrated in colour*
Serves 12.
3g fibre/190 calories per portion.

Imperial (Metric)

4 oz (100g) unsalted butter or
  polyunsaturated margarine
3 oz (75g) clear honey
4 free-range eggs, separated
2 oz (50g) wholemeal flour
4 oz (100g) wholemeal semolina
1 teaspoonful baking powder
4 oz (100g) ground coconut

American

½ cupful unsalted butter or
  polyunsaturated margarine
¼ cupful clear honey
4 free-range eggs, separated
½ cupful wholewheat flour
1 cupful wholewheat semolina
1 teaspoonful baking soda
1¼ cupsful ground coconut

1. Beat together the butter or margarine and honey until light and fluffy.

2. Gradually add egg yolks.

3. Sieve the flour, semolina and baking powder together and return bran from sieve to flour. Fold into the creamed mixture.

4. Stir in the coconut.

5. Whisk the egg whites until firm enough to hold stiff peaks. Fold into the mixture with a metal spoon.

6. Pour into a lightly oiled and lined cake tin and bake at 350°F/180°C (Gas Mark 4) for 40 minutes until golden brown and firm to the touch.

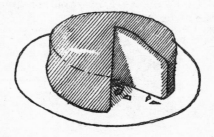

CINNAMON SWIRLS

Serves 4.
5g fibre/270 calories per portion.

Imperial (Metric)	American
1½ lb (¾ kilo) sweet potato	1½ pounds sweet potato
1 oz (25g) unsalted butter or polyunsaturated margarine	2½ tablespoonsful unsalted butter or polyunsaturated margarine
2 fl oz (60ml) soured cream	⅓ cupful soured cream
1 tablespoonful honey	1 tablespoonful honey
1 teaspoonful ground cinnamon	1 teaspoonful ground cinnamon
1 free-range egg yolk, beaten	1 free-range egg yolk, beaten
1 orange	1 orange
1 tablespoonful skimmed milk	1 tablespoonful skimmed milk

1. Scrub the potatoes and bake, unpeeled, at 400°F/200°C (Gas Mark 6) for 1 hour. Remove from oven, cut in half and scoop out all the flesh.

2. Pass flesh through a sieve or liquidize and mix with fat, cream, honey, cinnamon and egg yolk.

3. Add grated rind of orange and turn the mixture into a piping bag with a ½ in. (1cm) star nozzle.

4. Pipe rounds onto a lightly oiled baking tray and glaze with milk. Bake at 400°F/200°C (Gas Mark 6) for 20 minutes.

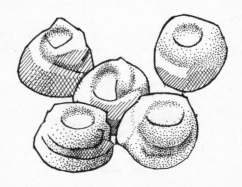

DATE FLAPJACKS *Illustrated in colour*
Makes 8.
3½g fibre/240 calories per flapjack.

Imperial (Metric)
4 oz (100g) polyunsaturated
   margarine
2 oz (50g) clear honey
½ lb (¼ kilo) rolled oats
4 oz (100g) dates, chopped
4 tablespoonsful water
½ lb (¼ kilo) cooking apple, grated
   but not peeled

American
½ cupful polyunsaturated margarine
2½ tablespoonsful clear honey
2 cupsful rolled oats
1 cupful dates, chopped
⅓ cupful water
1½ cupsful cooking apple, grated
   but not peeled

1. Melt the margarine and honey in a saucepan.

2. Stir in the oats. Set on one side.

3. Place the dates and water in another pan and cook to a soft pulp.

4. Add the apple to the dates and cook for a further few minutes.

5. Place half of the oat mixture in the bottom of a lightly oiled small cake tin.

6. Top with the date mixture and place the rest of the oats on the top. Level the mixture.

7. Bake at 350°F/180°C (Gas Mark 4) for 30 minutes, until golden brown.

8. Remove from the oven and mark into fingers. Do not remove from the tin until cold. Before removing re-cut sections.

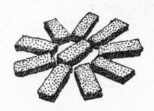

CARROT AND BANANA BREAD
Serves 8.
4g fibre/300 calories per portion.

Imperial (Metric)
10 oz (300g) wholemeal flour
1 teaspoonful baking powder
1/2 teaspoonful mixed spice
4 oz (100g) unsalted butter or
   polyunsaturated margarine
4 oz (100g) Barbados sugar
2 free-range eggs
1 large banana, mashed
1 large carrot, grated
1 oz (25g) sesame seeds

American
2 1/2 cupsful wholewheat flour
1 teaspoonful baking soda
1/2 teaspoonful mixed spice
1/2 cupful unsalted butter or
   polyunsaturated margarine
2/3 cupful Barbados sugar
2 free-range eggs
1 large banana, mashed
1 large carrot, grated
2 tablespoonsful sesame seeds

1. Sieve the flour, baking powder and spice into a bowl.

2. In another bowl cream the margarine and sugar until light and fluffy.

3. Beat the eggs and gradually add to the margarine mixture.

4. Stir in the banana, carrot and sesame seeds.

5. Fold in the flour. Turn into a lightly oiled loaf tin and bake at 350°F/180°C (Gas Mark 4) for 45 minutes.

INDEX